Pathophysiology, Homeos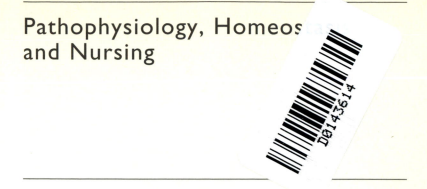
and Nursing

Nursing students quite often find it difficult to relate what they learn about normal and abnormal physiology to patient care. In this useful text Roger Watson and Tonks N. Fawcett clearly explain:

- the concept of homeostasis;
- the relevance of physiology to common disorders;
- the patient's response to these disorders;
- the appropriate nursing responses.

Each chapter is presented in a standard format with a brief outline of the relevant normal physiology and how homeostatic mechanisms usually cope. The book explains what the patient with a specific disorder feels like and why, and the reader is clearly instructed as to what nursing action to take.

Pathophysiology, Homeostasis and Nursing shows how understanding physiology can improve nursing care. It covers the main issues that relate to basic observations and includes questions to help readers test their knowledge as they go along. The book is an accessible, concise text for health care students, particularly nurses.

Roger Watson is Professor of Nursing in the School of Nursing, Social Work and Applied Health Studies, University of Hull, and **Tonks N. Fawcett** is Senior Lecturer for Nursing Studies at the School of Health and Wellbeing, College of Humanities and Social Science, University of Edinburgh.

Routledge Essentials for Nurses

Edited by Robert Newell, *University of Bradford*, and
David Thompson, *Chinese University of Hong Kong*

The series covers four key areas of nursing:

- core theoretical studies
- psychological and physical care
- nurse education
- new directions in nursing and health care

Written by experienced practitioners and teachers, books in the series encourage a critical approach to nursing concepts and show how research findings are relevant to nursing practice.

Also in the series:

Nursing Theories and Models
Hugh McKenna

Nursing Perspectives on Quality of Life
Peter Draper

Education for Patients and Clients
Vivien Coates

Caring for People in Pain
Bryn D. Davis

Body Image and Disfigurement Care
Robert Newell

Design and Analysis of Clinical Nursing Research Studies
Colin R. Martin and David R. Thompson

Sociology and Nursing
Peter Morrall

Pathophysiology, Homeostasis and Nursing

Roger Watson and
Tonks N. Fawcett

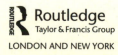
Routledge
Taylor & Francis Group

LONDON AND NEW YORK

First published 2003
by Routledge
11 New Fetter Lane, London EC4P 4EE

Simultaneously published in the USA and Canada
by Routledge
29 West 35th Street, New York, NY 10001

Routledge is an imprint of the Taylor & Francis Group

Typeset in Times New Roman by
Newgen Imaging Systems (P) Ltd, Chennai, India
Printed and bound in Great Britain by
TJ International Ltd, Padstow, Cornwall

British Library Cataloguing in Publication Data
A catalogue record for this book is available
from the British Library

Library of Congress Cataloging in Publication Data
Watson, Roger, 1955–
    Pathophysiology, homeostasis and nursing / Roger Watson and
Tonks N. Fawcett.
        p. cm. (Core theoretical studies)
    Includes bibliographical references and index.
        1. Homeostasis. 2. Human physiology. 3. Physiology, Pathological.
4. Nursing. I. Fawcett, Josephine N. II. Title. III. Series.

RT9.W38 2003
616.07–dc21   2003046660

ISBN 0–415–27549–0 (Hbk)
ISBN 0–415–27550–4 (Pbk)

Contents

Preface

Nursing students often find the biological sciences component of their educational programmes challenging and the reasons for this are manifold. They include such things as a poor level of science education at school, the teaching of biological science at university by non-nurse specialists who struggle to convey the relevance of the subject to students and the teaching of biological sciences by nurses who are not adequately prepared in terms of their own biological education. Students who struggle with this essential aspect of their education are, arguably, more likely to struggle with more clinically oriented aspects of their course. They are unlikely, fully, to understand what their patients are experiencing as a result of a disorder such as preexia, finding it difficult to make the links between pathophysiology, homeostasis and nursing care. Thereby, they are likely to be less effective at alleviating suffering and explaining illness to patients.

There are a considerable number of textbooks that are used to convey the biological sciences, in particular anatomy and physiology, to nursing students. However, these are either pitched too high for many entrants to nurse education courses or they are pitched too low to take students very far into their course. In addition, many of the textbooks most commonly used by nursing students are not specifically written for nurses. They, therefore, contain much information not directly relevant to their educational or practice requirements.

There are some notable exceptions in terms of textbooks that are written by nurses or designed, specifically, to convey the essential aspects of anatomy and physiology that nursing students require. Nevertheless, the main thrust of these texts – while they do contain clinically relevant material – is to convey the normal aspects of physiology in preparation for learning about disorders. Since *Pathology and Patient Care* (Jackson 1982) went out of print, there are no concise texts that convey how disorder is expressed in physiological or pathophysiological terms in such a way that students learn to link directly their understanding of normal physiology with the signs and symptoms that patients experience. Texts purporting to do this are not usually written for nurses and tend also to cover a great deal of normal physiology making them large texts with much material that is not directly relevant or is repeated. Specific pathology texts are usually too dry and detailed. However, there are some more recent textbooks, aimed at medical students, which introduce pathophysiology at an appropriate level but which do not include patient care relevant to nursing.

This text will be aimed at both pre-registration diploma and undergraduate nurses and is intended to be neither a comprehensive book on pathology nor a comprehensive book on patient care. Rather, it is intended to present some common disorders that will be encountered by nurses in almost any setting and to make explicit the relevance of physiology to common disorders and to patient care. As such, this is a companion text and readers are referred to other more detailed texts listed at the end of this preface. Many of these books have been referred to in the preparation of this book. In writing the present book we are not being critical of any of the texts listed. We were, however, aiming to produce a text that could be read in isolation from any set curriculum. We hope that nursing students, pre- and post-registration, undergraduate and postgraduate, will enjoy reading this book – perhaps on the train or in bed – as an introduction to the life sciences in nursing or just as a reference book that helps to put more detailed knowledge into place. If nothing else, we hope this text will go some way to helping the reader gain an understanding of the processes in their own body.

Material in the chapters will be presented in a standard format with a brief outline of the relevant normal physiology and how homeostatic mechanisms normally operate. Patient responses – what they experience – will be included and nursing interventions will be specific. Chapters will be preceded by learning outcomes and will be followed by a few short test questions related to the contents.

The following books were consulted in the preparation of this text:

Alexander M, Fawcett JN and Runciman P (2000) *Nursing Practice: Hospital and Home – the Adult.* Churchill Livingstone, Edinburgh.

Blows WT (2001) *The Biological Basis of Nursing: Clinical Observations.* Routledge, London.

Christiansen JL and Grzybowski JM (1993) *Biology of Aging.* Mosby, St Louis.

Clancy J and McVicar AJ (1998) *Nursing Care: a Homeostatic Casebook.* Arnold, London.

Clancy J and McVicar AJ (2002) *Physiology and Anatomy: A Homeostatic Approach*, 2nd edn. Arnold, London.

Clancy J, McVicar AJ and Baird N (2002) *Perioperative Practice: Fundamentals of Homeostasis*. Routledge, London.

Higgins C (2000) *Understanding Laboratory Investigations: A Text for Nurses and Healthcare Professionals*. Blackwell, Oxford.

Hinchliff S, Montague S and Watson R (1996) *Physiology for Nursing Practice*, 2nd edn. Baillière Tindall, London.

Marieb EN (2001) *Human Anatomy and Physiology*, 5th edn. Addison Wesley Longman, San Francisco.

McGhee M (2000) *A Guide to Laboratory Investigations*, 3rd edn. Radcliffe Medical Press, Oxford.

Martini FH (2000) *Fundamentals of Anatomy and Physiology*, 5th edn. Prentice Hall, New Jersey.

Phillips J, Muray P and Kirk P (2001) *The Biology of Disease*. Blackwell, Oxford.

Tortora GJ and Grabowski SR (2003) *Principles of Anatomy and Physiology*, 10th edn. John Wiley and Sons Inc, New York.

Walsh M (2002) *Watson's Clinical Nursing and Related Sciences*, 6th edn. Baillière Tindall, London.

Watson R (1999) *Essential Science for Nursing Students: An Introductory Text*. Baillière Tindall, London.

Watson R (2000) *Anatomy and Physiology for Nurses*, 11th edn. Baillière Tindall, London.

Acknowledgements

Figures 1.1, 2.1, 2.2, 4.2, 4.3, 6.1, 6.2 and 7.1 reprinted from *Anatomy and Physiology for Nurses*, 11th edn, Watson, R. © 2000 Elsevier Inc.

Figures 7.2, 7.3 and 8.2 reprinted from *Nursing Practice Hospital and Home*, 2nd edn, Alexander, M., Fawcett, J. and Runciman, P. © 2000 Elsevier Ltd.

Table 7.1 reprinted from *Watson's Clinical Nursing and Related Science*, 6th edn, Walsh M. © 2002 Elsevier Ltd.

Figures 3.3, 3.4, 5.1, 5.2 and 8.1 and Tables 8.1 and 8.2 reprinted from *Physiology for Nursing Practice*, 2nd edn, Hinchcliff, S., Montagure, S. and Watson, R. © 1999 Elsevier Ltd.

Chapter 1

Introduction

Aim

To provide an overview of homeostasis.

Learning outcomes

This introductory chapter will enable the reader to:

- gain an appreciation of the nature of homeostasis;
- understand the purpose of homeostasis;
- identify the components of homeostasis;
- understand some examples of homeostasis;
- understand the effect of ageing on homeostasis;
- demonstrate the relevance of homeostasis to nursing practice.

Introduction

The body works because it is able to maintain a constant internal environment. The fact that the body has a constant internal environment was first observed by the French physiologist Claude Bernard (1813–78), who observed 'it is the constancy of the internal environment which is the condition of free and independent life. All vital mechanisms, however varied they may be, have only one object, that of preserving constant the conditions of life in the internal environment.' The process whereby this constant internal environment is maintained is called homeostasis and this concept, first described in 1932 by Walter Cannon, will be referred to frequently throughout this book. This chapter is designed to give an overview of the reasons why homeostasis is important, what it achieves and how it is achieved.

The maintenance of homeostasis provides the basic necessities of health. Deviations in health commonly result in deviations from homeostasis and also result from deviations in homeostasis. The process of homeostasis is self-regulating and every system of the body is involved in this regulation. In fact, maintaining homeostasis is undoubtedly the most important physiological function of the body.

Homeostasis aims to maintain a constant internal environment in order that all the cells of the body can survive and function. Some cells will rapidly die if their conditions change even slightly with respect to pH, electrolyte balance, energy sources and temperature. By controlling the function of systems of the body such as the respiratory and renal systems, homeostasis achieves constancy with respect to the optimal conditions for cell survival and function. Therefore, homeostasis regulates the levels of oxygen, carbon dioxide, electrolytes, acid and alkali, glucose and hormones in our blood. In addition, homeostasis regulates our body temperature and blood pressure.

Why do we need homeostasis?

We need homeostasis because our body constantly faces changes that threaten to disrupt its function by preventing cells and thereby tissues and organs from functioning as well as they should. For example, we regularly and frequently subject our bodies to many changes in condition, for example, environmental and nutritional, which would be life-threatening were it not for the process of homeostasis. In fact, so effective are the processes of homeostasis that we are hardly aware of such changes in condition – unless they become very extreme. We move from warm to cold environments and, albeit that we take behavioural measures such as putting on or removing clothing, the body is still subject to changes in environmental temperature that have to be very wide before serious problems or even discomfort arises. We require a constant level of glucose in our blood in order for our body to function. This is especially true of our brains, which are entirely dependent upon glucose as a source of energy. However, despite snacks, we usually only eat substantial amounts two or three times daily. Likewise, the body requires water, which is one of its major components (approximately 70 per cent) to function. However, we do not drink constantly but take drinks with meals and at other times throughout the day. The above examples illustrate what homeostasis achieves. The mechanisms will be explained in more detail in subsequent chapters but in the case of body temperature, despite changing environmental temperature and the changes we impose upon ourselves, the core temperature of the body is kept constant by homeostasis and this is achieved through mechanisms that show that we can either conserve or lose heat. Similarly, the body can conserve or lose water, as it requires in order to keep body water constant and, in fact, this mechanism is tied in to the mechanism for regulating body temperature. In the case of blood glucose, the body is able to remove glucose from the blood to be stored elsewhere in the body following a meal. However, as time from the last meal increases and blood glucose tends to fall, there are mechanisms that remove glucose from storage and into the blood in order to keep the blood levels constant until the next meal.

How does homeostasis work?

Homeostasis is a dynamic system that is able to help the body to respond to changing conditions. The outcome of homeostasis is that there is no significant change in the internal environment of the body but this does not mean that nothing is happening. In order for a system to be dynamic and responsive to change, the system has to be able to detect the changes that are taking place, it must then be able to act in such a way that the change is rectified, and such a system needs to be controlled. In fact, all of the components of a homeostatic system have been described above; a homeostatic system must have a detector, an effector and a control centre (Figure 1.1). A good analogy is driving a car and trying to keep it at a constant speed: the detector of speed is the speedometer and the effector, whereby speed is regulated, is the accelerator pedal, which can be depressed or raised in order to make the car go faster or slower, respectively. The control centre is you, the driver, who senses that speed is changing by reading the speedometer and then responds by changing the speed through the action of your feet on the accelerator pedal.

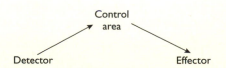

Figure 1.1 The components of a homeostatic system.

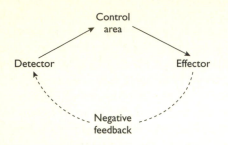

Figure 1.2 The components of a homeostatic system including negative feedback.

Negative feedback

The above analogy of homeostasis also demonstrates the mechanism by which most homeostatic systems work: negative feedback. In a negative feedback system, the detection that the system is moving away from homeostasis results in an action taking place, which negates the movement away from homeostasis. In the case of the car, for example, if it is going too fast then your foot is taken off the pedal until the car slows down. Once the car has slowed down, it is detected that a constant speed has been reached and you try to keep to that speed by making further small adjustments to the accelerator pedal. This also illustrates another aspect of negative feedback; in other words, the corrective action stops once homeostasis has been achieved (Figure 1.2). In reality, just as in the car driving analogy, the body is constantly making small adjustments to maintain homeostasis, of which we are largely unaware, and only occasionally do large adjustments have to be made under exceptional circumstances.

What are the challenges to homeostasis?

Homeostasis keeps a number of body parameters within a reasonably narrow range through its ability to detect movement beyond or outside these normal parameters and make the necessary corrections. However, the capacity of homeostasis, while perfectly adequate for normal daily life in a temperate climate, is not infinite. The body can encounter conditions where homeostasis is challenged either through the rate of change of circumstances or the extremes to which they are taken. Returning to the analogy with the motor car: if the accelerator pedal is held down hard without being raised then irreparable damage will be done to the engine. Conversely, if the brake pedal is held down without being raised then the car will stop. Neither of these end points is compatible with the 'homeostatic' state of constant speed to which it aspired. Extending the analogy, if the car suddenly collides with a wall it will also stop – dramatically – and also sees an end to the 'homeostatic' state that was being aimed for.

The body can be challenged suddenly by situations that may significantly challenge homeostasis. An example of this is trauma. In trauma, caused by sudden and severe damage to the body (e.g. if you were in the car that crashed into the wall), the body can lose large amounts of blood and enter a state of 'shock', which homeostasis cannot compensate for as the loss of blood is too severe. Disease can also challenge homeostasis in many ways. If we become infected by a microorganism, one response of our body is to raise the core temperature to help the action of the cells and enzymes that help the body to defend itself against infection. This raised body temperature is called pyrexia. The body suppresses the normal homeostatic mechanisms, such as perspiring, in order to conspire with the pyrexia and reaches a new steady, if not strictly speaking, homeostatic state. However, the rise in body temperature can be extreme in some circumstances and in some susceptible individuals and can lead to damage to the body and even death. In such cases, the homeostatic mechanism for maintaining body temperature has been challenged and compromised beyond its ability to respond sufficiently.

Another circumstance under which homeostasis is challenged is during surgical or medical interventions. Surgery, while it is carried out with great care and precision, inflicts planned trauma on the body and alters the state of the body in such a way that homeostatic mechanisms may have to work hard both during and after surgery in order to keep a constant internal environment. For example, surgery can lead to blood loss, lowered body temperature, a wound that must heal and the potential for infection – all at once. These may be outside of the range within which homeostasis works and additional measures may be required in order to compensate. Medical procedures and treatment interventions may lead to disturbances in homeostasis, which may be extreme, requiring additional measures to help. For example, a side-effect of some necessary antibiotics may be diarrhoea leading to fluid loss, some analgesic medicines may result in gastric irritation and lead to internal bleeding and chemotherapy can reduce the body's natural immunity leaving it prone to infection. In a person who may already be ill the ability to cope with such challenges through normal homeostatic mechanisms may be further compromised.

Age and ageing

The disturbances to the body that challenge homeostasis described above are all abnormal due to the body being placed in extreme environmental situations, by trauma, disease or the outcome of medical or surgical intervention. However, there is a naturally occurring process that has a profound influence on homeostasis: the process of ageing.

The outward signs and other consequences of ageing are well catalogued: for example, loss of elasticity in the skin, reduced joint flexibility, bone loss and muscle atrophy. However, how the process of ageing takes place and, especially, why it takes place is poorly understood. One consequence of ageing is a reduced ability to carry out homeostasis; for example, a reduced detection of such things as fluid loss and temperature changes, particularly hypothermia, which are potentially life-threatening for some older people.

Older people are perfectly able to carry out homeostasis under what could be described as normal circumstances. They are less able, however, to withstand deviations from normal and, as indicated above, are less able to adapt to extremes of temperature. Particularly when illness intervenes, the inability to withstand the consequences of, for example, dehydration increases the vulnerability of older patients. Most of the systems of the body are affected to some extent by the process of ageing and although there is considerable excess capacity that can be called upon in times of biological stress, the capacity of older people to withstand and adapt to biological stress is reduced. For example, the blood vessels of older people are less responsive to circulating catecholamines – hormones that alter the diameter of blood vessels, amongst other things – and thereby older people adapt less readily to changes in blood pressure. This can manifest itself in quite serious conditions such as postural hypotension where the cardiovascular system of an older person, upon standing up, does not adjust by the necessary vasoconstriction, to ensure cerebral perfusion resulting in dizziness and fainting.

The reduced detection of temperature changes will be compounded by such social circumstances as poverty and loneliness where the combination of poorly heated homes, inactivity and an insensitivity to their falling body temperature can result in a dramatically reduced core body temperature, which, without intervention, becomes life-threatening.

Older people are more prone to infections due to the immune system, our means of defence against infection, becoming less efficient. In addition, with the failing homeostatic mechanisms, infection in older people is often not accompanied by pyrexia and this may result in, not only a reduced efficiency of the body's response to infection, but also a less obvious manifestation of infectious disorder for others, relatives, nurses or doctors, to observe.

While most systems of the body do have considerable excess capacity and the reductions with age are not really significant, the renal system undergoes marked reduction in capacity with age and this is manifested as a reduced ability to filter blood by the kidneys. Clearly, this is not a problem under normal circumstances but in illness where drugs are prescribed this can be a problem for older people. Most drugs are excreted at the kidneys into the urine and a reduction in filtration will mean that less of the drug is excreted from the body. A problem arises here due to the fact that older people are less responsive to some drugs and there is a tendency to increase the dose of some drugs in order to get the desired effect. However, without due care and attention an older person can begin to suffer from their medication rather than benefit from it and the maxim for prescribers is to lower the dose of the drug and lengthen the period between taking the drug for older people.

Homeostasis: the working parts

An outline of how homeostasis works was given above along with the vital components: detector, effector and control centre in abstract terms followed by some real physiological examples. However, the components of homeostasis differ between systems and there are specific detectors and effectors for each system. Whilst this is not exclusive, it can more or less be taken for granted that the control centre for a homeostatic system lies in the brain – often in a region of the brain called the hypothalamus. Specific examples will be provided throughout the rest of the book but two simple examples, to which reference has already been made above, provided in more detail should help in the application of general principles to specific systems.

Blood pressure is an example of a system that is regulated homeostatically. The control centre is the hypothalamus and changes in blood pressure are detected by specialised nerve endings called baroreceptors (baro = pressure) in specific regions of the cardiovascular system. The baroreceptors respond to stretch and as the blood pressure increases in the cardiovascular system they are stretched and send signals to the control centre in the hypothalamus that pressure in the cardiovascular system is increasing. The response of the control centre in the hypothalamus is to send signals to the cardiovascular system through nerves and hormones (blood-borne chemicals), which lower the blood pressure. We see, in the regulation of blood pressure, the combined action of nerves and hormones in the control of a system. The nerves take signals from the cardiovascular system to the brain (an afferent pathway) and the brain then responds by nervous and hormonal pathways (an efferent pathway) back to the cardiovascular system.

Another good example of homeostasis is the control of water balance in the body. If we do not drink enough, receptors (osmoreceptors and thirst receptors) in the brain are stimulated and we are stimulated, on the one hand, to drink more, which is a behavioural response mediated through the nervous system. However, a hormone is also released from the brain (antidiuretic hormone), which reduces the production of urine and thereby reduces the loss of water from the body. By this point is should be apparent that homeostasis is a process that is constantly working to maintain the stable internal environment of the body, it is composed of common components and works through the co-operation of nerves and hormones, usually with the brain in control.

Nursing and homeostasis

A significant, but by no means exclusive, part of the nursing role is compensating for disturbances of homeostasis. It could be said, in one sense, therefore, that where homeostasis ends, nursing begins. Nurses are often involved in helping the sick and often older individuals to overcome the effects of illness: trauma and surgery, which can all leave the body in homeostatic imbalance. The remainder of the book will provide more detailed explanations of the physiological mechanisms at work and the rationale behind nursing actions but, briefly, it is worth outlining some of the main features of nursing care in this area as a framework for subsequent chapters.

Illness, trauma and surgery can lead to several detrimental outcomes such as raised body temperature, dehydration and malnutrition, all of which represent homeostatic imbalance for the patient. Physical nursing care of patients seeks to compensate, for example, for raised body temperature by helping the body to lose heat by removing clothing, bathing in tepid water or administering drugs such as paracetamol, which can reset the imbalance in the homeostatic system that is regulating body temperature. If a patient is dehydrated then the nurse has a responsibility to monitor this and to help restore fluid levels in the body by encouraging the patient to drink more or by administering intravenous fluids in more severe cases. However, this physical imperative is embedded in holistic care, which seeks to understand the patient's physical, psychological and social well-being such that the nurse understands each patient's unique situation and supports physical interventions with interpersonal means whereby the reality of homeostatic imbalances is fully understood.

Conclusion

In order to give good nursing care, which compensates for homeostatic imbalance, the nurse first needs, broadly, to understand the concept homeostasis. This has been the function of this introductory chapter. Based on an understanding of homeostasis the nurse can then know what to expect under certain circumstances, for example, following trauma or surgery or in old age. Arguably, these things can be learned by rote but how much more meaningful will be the learning if an understanding is gained of the underlying physiological principles. How much more meaningful will then be the recognition of the signs and symptoms which indicate that problems may be present and how much discerning will be our plan of care.

The purpose of this book is to demonstrate the importance of understanding the general principles of homeostasis and homeostatic imbalance that result in from disease or disorder. It is not medicine but a means whereby some of the essential nursing knowledge and skilled interventions, in partnership with other members of the health care team, can be understood.

Questions

1   Can you explain what homeostasis is?
2   How does homeostasis work?
3   What would the consequences be for the body without homeostasis?
4   What part do nerves and hormones play in homeostasis?
5   Can you explain what negative feedback is?
6   How is homeostasis affected by ageing?
7   Giving examples, identify specific nursing interventions that may be required should specific homeostatic mechanisms fail.

Chapter 2

Fluid balance

Aim

To gain an understanding of the importance of water in the body.

Learning outcomes

This chapter will enable the reader to:

- understand the nature of water;
- describe and explain the principles of diffusion and osmosis;
- explain transport mechanisms across membranes;
- understand and describe oedema and lymphoedema;
- recognise the importance of documenting all fluid gains and losses in patients whose fluid homeostasis is disturbed.

Introduction

The main fluid in the body is water and the importance of water in the body can be realised if we consider that 70 per cent of the body is composed of water. Water is found inside cells and outside cells in the plasma and in the fluid between cells, the interstitial fluid. Water is described as the universal solvent because a large variety of substances dissolve in it and this is a large part of the function of water in the body. For example, the blood carries a wide range of substances dissolved in the plasma from simple ionic compounds such as electrolytes to relatively complex molecules such as hormones.

Water bathes every cell and tissue and organ of the body and the cells of the body are dependent upon their water content to maintain structure and function. The water surrounding the cells and tissues serves several functions such as providing protection in the brain, giving form and support to body structures such as the eye, bringing nutrients to the cell and removing waste products. Water also plays a part in control of the cells and tissues where it acts as a medium for chemical messengers such as hormones and neurotransmitters. It can be seen, therefore, that any disturbance to water homeostasis, or fluid balance, can have potentially very serious consequences for all the organs and systems of the body.

What is water?

Body water is distributed between two major compartments, the intracellular fluid (ICF) and the extracellular fluid (ECF). The ICF comprises about 50 per cent of body water and the ECF is comprised of the watery component of the blood, the plasma and the water that is found between cells, the interstitial fluid. The nature of the fluid compartments of the body and exchanges between them are largely determined by the nature of water; therefore, the physical chemistry of water will be briefly considered before moving on to the physiological aspects of fluid balance.

Water is a polar molecule composed of two atoms of hydrogen covalently bonded to one molecule of oxygen. A covalent molecule is one where a pair of electrons is shared and the water molecule is described as being polar because the two ends of the water molecule carry slight opposite charges and this polarity is what gives water its unique properties (Figure 2.1). The polarity arises because the pairs of electrons in the covalent bonds of water are unevenly distributed between the two atoms that form the bond: the electrons are more

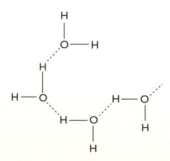

Figure 2.1 Diagrammatic representation of hydrogen bonding in water. The broken lines are the weak interactions between the oxygen and hydrogen atoms.

attracted to the oxygen end of the bond giving the oxygen atom a slight negative charge and the hydrogen atoms a slight positive charge.

The polar nature of water provides a chemical coherence between the water molecules called hydrogen bonding: the slightly negatively charged oxygen atom attracts the slightly positively charged hydrogen atoms and, thus, each water molecule is slightly attracted to those around it and the hydrogen bonding leads to surface tension. Of more importance, the mutual attraction between molecules of water gives it its liquid physical state without which the water would simply evaporate and there would be no rivers, lakes and seas. Life as we know it would be an impossible proposition.

The polar nature of water, in addition to its unique structural features, also provides it with it solvent properties; it is called the 'universal solvent'. Water acts as a solvent by enabling the breakdown of large complex structures that are held together by relatively weak forces into their constituent molecules. Excellent examples of substances that water can dissolve, and are thereby described as solutes, are common salt (sodium chloride) and common sugar (sucrose). The molecules of sodium chloride are held together in crystalline form by ionic bonds that result from the electrostatic attraction between the negatively charged chlorine and the positively charged sodium. When the two constituent atoms come together an electron is lost from sodium and gained by chlorine. In the case of sucrose, the polarised sucrose molecules are attracted to water molecules by hydrogen bonds. The function of water, in dissolving substances such as sucrose and salt is, as a result of its polar nature, to surround charged or slightly charged molecules so as to neutralise their charges and, thereby, prevent the attraction between the molecules. The process can be reversed by removing the water, for example, by evaporation.

Diffusion

If a small soluble crystal, for example, blue copper sulphate which is easily seen, is dropped into water, the crystal will immediately begin to dissolve and this may be observed by the gradual spread of blue colouration throughout the water. Eventually, the crystal will disappear and the water will be a uniform blue colour and this has arisen due to a process called diffusion. The water molecules are in constant movement as they form and re-form hydrogen bonds between the water molecules and this process moves the molecules of copper sulphate throughout the whole volume of water. Obviously, the process can be speeded up by increasing the movement of the water molecules by stirring the water or heating it, concepts we are familiar with through the process of making tea or coffee. The greater the amount of a substance we dissolve in water the more concentrated the solution will be; in other words, there will be a greater number of molecules of the solute in every given volume of the solvent.

While the movement of molecules in the water is entirely random, diffusion is not without direction as the tendency is for molecules to move, or diffuse, from areas of high concentration to areas of lower concentration – that is, down a concentration gradient – and this is demonstrated by the eventual movement of the blue colour of copper sulphate throughout the whole volume of water. This aspect of diffusion is important to appreciate, as it will be referred to below.

Water and membranes

Water is able to cross some membranes while molecules such as sugar and salt are retained. These membranes are described as being semi-permeable membranes. The movement of water across semi-permeable membranes is called osmosis and this is a crucial process in the body because it is by osmosis that water moves in and out of cells. Osmosis is described as the movement of water across a semi-permeable membrane from a region of high concentration of water to a region of low concentration of water. It is best demonstrated by considering two solutions of salt separated by a semi-permeable membrane. If the solution of salt on one side of the membrane is more concentrated than the solution on the other side then the more concentrated salt solution contains a lower concentration of water. The result, due to osmosis, is that water will move from the less concentrated salt solution to the more concentrated salt solution until the concentration of salt – and thereby water – on either side of the membrane is the same; that is, they are isotonic (Figure 2.2).

The extent to which a solution will cause water to move into it through a semi-permeable membrane is called osmotic potential. The fluids of the body, inside cells, in the bloodstream and between cells all have the same osmotic potential and the maintenance of this osmotic potential in these fluids is a major homeostatic function that will be described below. However, the devastating effects of not being able to maintain a constant internal environment with respect to osmotic potential can be demonstrated by changing the osmotic potential of a solution containing red blood cells. If the solution in which the cells are suspended is of the same concentration as the fluid inside the cells then the cells will

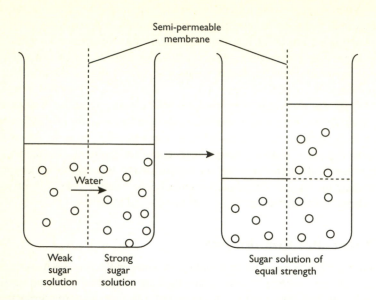

Figure 2.2 Diagram to show osmosis.

maintain their normal shape, size and appearance. If the solution is made hypertonic, fluid will move – by osmosis – out of the cells and they will shrink, a process called crenation. If the solution in which the cells are suspended is made hypotonic then fluid will move into the cells and they will swell. If the solution is very hypotonic the cells will eventually burst, a process called haemolysis. It is possible to imagine the dire consequences of this happening in the human bloodstream: the red blood cells would no longer be able to carry out their function of transporting blood gases. Fortunately, this is unlikely to occur in the body due to homeostasis.

Molecules and membranes

Cells are surrounded by a semi-permeable membrane composed of a unique combination of lipids and protein called the plasma membrane. The plasma membrane is responsible for controlling what enters and leaves the cell, in addition to some other functions such as recognition of other cells. This section will consider the movement of molecules, other than water, across membranes as this is also crucial to the homeostasis of fluids in the body. When a molecule in solution encounters a cell membrane, the molecule, depending upon its properties, may be able to cross the membrane relatively easily or may not be able to cross the membrane at all. The properties of the molecule that will dictate the ease with which it crosses the membrane will be its size, whether or not it is charged (hydrophilic, i.e. water 'loving') or lipid (hydrophobic, i.e. water 'hating') in nature. Essentially, large hydrophilic molecules cross membranes less easily than small hydrophobic molecules. However, relatively large hydrophilic molecules such as glucose can sometimes still cross the cell membrane as will be explained below. Whether or not a particular molecule crosses the cell membrane into the cell will largely depend on whether the molecule is useful to the cell or not.

There are three ways in which molecules may pass through membranes and these are diffusion, facilitated diffusion and active transport. Standard physiology texts, some of which are referred to in the reading list for this book, offer excellent explanations and examples of these processes, which will simply be compared and contrasted here (Table 2.1). The process of diffusion in solution was described above and the process of diffusion of substances across cell membranes is similar in that the diffusion takes place – and can only take place – down a concentration gradient. In other words, the solute that is able to diffuse across the plasma membrane must be in a higher concentration on one side of the membrane that the other and it will diffuse from the more concentrated solution to the less concentrated solution until the concentration on either side is the same. In physiology, the concentrations of

Table 2.1 Mechanisms of transport across the plasma membrane

Mechanism	Characteristics
Diffusion	Can only occur down a concentration gradient, no energy required and only particles small enough to cross the plasma membrane will diffuse across.
Facilitated transport	Can only occur down a concentration gradient, no energy required but large particles can cross the plasma membrane at specialised sites, or carriers, on the membrane.
Active transport	Can occur against a concentration gradient and carrier sites and energy is required.

solutes on either side of a plasma membrane are never the same as the substances which are removed by metabolism inside the cell, thereby reducing the concentration and ensuring that more of the substance diffuses in. Or, on the other hand, some substances such as waste products of cell metabolism are constantly removed from the fluid surrounding the cell by the bloodstream. A good example of two substances that diffuse freely across the plasma membrane are oxygen and carbon dioxide and this will be considered in detail later with respect to the control of the respiratory system. For the present purposes it is sufficient to note that oxygen is constantly consumed by cells and, therefore, a concentration gradient exists between the outside and the inside of the plasma membrane. On the other hand, carbon dioxide is constantly being produced by cells and a concentration gradient also exists across the plasma membrane. It should be noted that the concentration gradients for oxygen and carbon dioxide run in different directions: the oxygen is more concentrated outside the cell and the carbon dioxide is more concentrated inside the cell. This illustrates the point that the concentration gradients refer to individual substances.

Facilitated diffusion, sometimes called facilitated transport, is similar to simple diffusion in that it can only operate down a concentration gradient. The difference between facilitated diffusion and simple diffusion is that facilitated diffusion takes place at specific sites on the plasma membrane that are designed to allow particular molecules to cross the membrane. Usually, these molecules will be too large or polar to cross by simple diffusion and one example is the sugar fructose, which is taken up into the cells of the small intestine by facilitated diffusion. The sites at which facilitated diffusion takes place are called carriers and these are proteins embedded in the plasma membrane and which penetrate from the outside of the membrane to the inside – to the cytoplasm. The difference between simple and facilitated diffusion may be observed by studying the uptake of substances into cells. In the case of simple diffusion, the rate of the process is infinite provided that the concentration gradient is maintained across the plasma membrane. However, in facilitated diffusion, the process is limited by the number of carrier sites on the plasma membrane. Once all the carrier sites are being used to transport a substance across the plasma membrane – that is, in chemical terms, they are saturated – the process cannot transport more rapidly regardless of the concentration gradient across the plasma membrane.

Active transport is an entirely different process from simple diffusion but is similar to facilitated diffusion in that it takes place at specific sites on the plasma membrane. However, unlike either simple diffusion or facilitated diffusion, active transport can transport substances up a concentration gradient and it achieves this by the expenditure of energy. Energy is usually supplied in the form of the ubiquitous high-energy molecule in the body, adenosine triphosphate (ATP), which is made using the calories in the food we eat. Active transport sites are enzymes that are capable of breaking down ATP, releasing the energy in the molecule and using it to transport molecules across the plasma membrane. Therefore, active transport is not dependent upon a concentration gradient in order to function but the rate at which it can work is limited, in the same way as for facilitated diffusion, by the number of carrier sites on the plasma membrane. Active transport is used to accumulate substances in cells that are large and polar but also essential. Thus, glucose is taken up by the cells of the small intestine by active transport and the tissues of the body have a high requirement for glucose. Another example of active transport is the sodium/potassium pump that is present in the plasma membrane of all cells. The sodium/potassium pump involves enzymes that break down ATP and uses this energy to pump sodium out of the cell and bring in potassium. Sodium and potassium in solution exist as ions; that is, they have a positive charge because they have lost an electron, usually to chlorine. By exchanging sodium ions for potassium ions the electrostatic charge across the membrane is maintained. This charge is very important to the function of nerve and muscle cells.

Fluid balance

We take fluids into the body in the food we eat and the drinks we consume. We can lose fluid from the body in the urine, from the lungs as we breathe, in perspiration, in faeces and we lose water, insensibly, from the surface of the skin. Under extreme circumstances, we can lose large amounts of fluid from the body in trauma where excessive bleeding is caused and following burns where the protective layer of the skin is lost and fluid exudes from the body. Under these circumstances, fluid taken by mouth may be insufficient or impossible and fluids must be administered by other routes, for example, intravenously, to compensate for the loss.

The body is considered to be in fluid balance when the intake of fluids into the body matches the output of fluids from the body, and the fluid compartments of the body have sufficient fluid. While the recommended daily intakes of fluid in temperate climates without taking exercise is approximately 1500 ml per day, there can be considerable variation around this in warmer climates and if a great deal of physical work is undertaken. The body can also maintain fluid balance across a wide range of intake by matching a very small input with a very small output – but only for a limited period – and vice versa.

The level of fluid in our body will be determined by how much we are eating and drinking, by our level of physical activity and the surrounding temperature. Fluid balance is also partly determined by our behaviour. The actual intake of fluid will be determined by how thirsty we become as there is a thirst centre in the hypothalamus of the brain that detects rising osmolarity in body fluids; an indicator that the concentration of solutes is increasing and the water content is falling. The resulting sensation of thirst will increase our tendency to drink. The detection of increased osmolarity by the hypothalamus also stimulates the release of an antidiuretic hormone, which acts on the renal system to conserve water in the body as explained below.

Fluid balance is also maintained in the body by the renal system, which can restrict the loss of fluid from the body or increase fluid loss, in the urine, as required. The renal system is comprised of two kidneys, two ureters and the urinary bladder. The kidneys are responsible for filtering the blood, reabsorbing essential components from the filtrate and then secreting substances in a continuous process. According to the fluid balance of the body, the kidneys can produce a dilute urine when fluid balance if positive (intake has exceeded output) and a concentrated urine when fluid balance is negative (output has exceeded intake). The bladder is responsible for the storage of urine until it is convenient to expel it from the body. The actual process that allows the kidney to vary the concentration of urine is beyond the scope of this book but the release of an antidiuretic hormone from the brain allows the kidneys to remove water from the urine that is being produced and return it to the body in the bloodstream. Thus, a homeostatic system is established with the detector being the brain, the effector being the kidney and the control centre, also in the brain, triggering the release of an antidiuretic hormone by the posterior pituitary gland.

Fluid imbalance

Having a severe excess of water in the body, while possible, is rare (although in clinical situations it may be possible to overload a patient with intravenous fluid). However, being depleted of water, or dehydrated, is more common. Dehydration due to loss of water on its own is rare but this will take place if we drink less water than we lose and also in extreme breathlessness whereby we lose water from the respiratory system. The outcome of losing excessive water from the body is that the concentration of electrolytes will increase in the body, particularly sodium, leading to hypernatraemia. Symptoms of hypernatraemia, due to the role that sodium plays in the stimulation and conduction in nerve and muscle tissue, include a rapid heart rate, confusion and even loss of consciousness. Usually, we lose both water and electrolytes from the body, for example, through excessive sweating or diarrhoea.

Exchange of fluid between compartments

The fluid in the body is constantly being exchanged between the fluid compartments of the body and these are the cells, the plasma and the interstitial fluids. Fluid is exchanged between the compartments by a combination of osmotic and hydrostatic pressure and healthy levels of fluid are maintained in each compartment as a result of the balance between these two forces. Osmotic pressure is highest in the plasma where the plasma proteins, which cannot normally pass out of the blood vessels, maintain it. At the same time, due to blood pressure on the blood vessels arising from the circulation of the blood, there is hydrostatic pressure: a pressure that tends to push fluid out of the blood vessels (Figure 2.3). The tendency, therefore, is for fluid to be pushed out of the blood by hydrostatic pressure and for fluid to be drawn back into the blood by osmotic pressure.

In health, due to the pumping action of the heart, the hydrostatic pressure is greater in the arterial side of the circulation than the venous side; in other words, it drops as the blood moves away from the heart. On

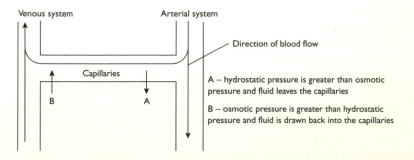

Figure 2.3 The movement of fluid in and out of the capillaries as a result of hydrostatic pressure and osmotic pressure.

the other hand, osmotic pressure remains constant throughout the cardiovascular system as the levels of plasma proteins remain constant. In fact, the hydrostatic pressure in the arterial side of the circulation exceeds the osmotic pressure and in the venous side of the circulation the osmotic pressure exceeds the hydrostatic pressure. The result is that there is a net movement of fluid out of the cardiovascular system at the arterial end of the circulation, across the capillaries, into the interstitial fluids where exchange of nutrients and waste products can take place. On the other hand, at the venous end of the capillaries there is a net movement of fluid back into the circulation. More fluid is pushed out of the circulation at the arterial end of the capillaries than is taken back up at the venous end and this excess of fluid enters the lymphatic capillaries and is returned directly to the circulation where the lymphatic system is joined to the cardiovascular system at the subclavian veins.

Oedema

Oedema is a condition, with many causes, which gives rise to excess interstitial fluid. The cardinal sign of oedema is swelling and it is affected by gravity, in other words, the fluid will find the lowest point in the body and is called dependent oedema. This is why it is common for the ankles to swell in cases of oedema.

Essentially, oedema arises due to an imbalance between the osmotic and hydrostatic pressures in the cardiovascular system. If osmotic pressure drops then it will rise and, likewise, if hydrostatic pressure in the venous system increases it will arise. A drop in osmotic pressure is unlikely but can rise in cases of prolonged protein-calorie malnutrition, or advanced liver failure, which lead to lowered levels of plasma proteins. Under these circumstances, there is insufficient osmotic pressure in the blood to draw fluid back into the cardiovascular system at the venous end of the capillaries and the lymphatic system cannot cope with the excess interstitial fluid.

Oedema more commonly arises when hydrostatic pressure at the venous end of the capillaries rises and this commonly results from heart failure, particularly of the right side of the heart (right atrium and right ventricle), which is responsible for collecting blood from the venous circulation and pumping it to the lungs. In heart failure, the ability of the heart to circulate the blood is impaired and hydrostatic pressure increases in the veins. This increase in hydrostatic pressure in the veins exceeds the osmotic pressure in the plasma and fluid remains in the interstitial fluid surrounding the capillaries. Oedema may be a minor problem to cope with in mild heart failure but can be more serious because it is preventing the exchange of nutrients and waste products between the blood and the tissues. The fluid is under the influence of gravity and if a person with heart failure is standing up the ankles will appear swollen. If they are sitting down with raised feet – a common way to relieve swollen ankles – the sacrum may swell. Ultimately, the only way to relieve the collection of excess fluid is to relieve the heart failure and this is achieved using drugs to remove excess fluid from the body (diuretics) and to help the heart to work more efficiently (inotropes).

Oedema can also occur if the left side of the heart fails to pump blood from the lungs into the systemic circulation. In this case, because there is no interstitial space in the lungs, the excess fluid leaks out into the alveoli of lungs where it prevents the exchange of oxygen and carbon dioxide between the alveoli and blood. This is called pulmonary oedema. If the failure of the left side of the heart is severe then the fluid can be coughed up as pink, frothy sputum, which is very characteristic of pulmonary oedema. The colour is due to the presence of red blood cells.

Oedema can also arise due to blockages in the lymphatic system, which may be caused by tumour obstruction in cancer or by certain types of parasitic disease. Under these circumstances, there is no change in either the osmotic pressure of the plasma or the hydrostatic pressure in the veins. The lymphatic system is unable to carry out its normal function of removing excess fluid from the interstitial tissues back into the bloodstream and the fluid accumulates in the areas that are served by the particular affected lymphatics. Lymphoedema, therefore, is often confined to one particular area of the body such as the limbs where the extent of the accumulation of tissue fluid can be extensive and distressing.

Conclusion

Water is essential for life and the body expends considerable energy, at rest, simply to maintain the balance of water between the extra- and intracellular compartments of the body. The balance and movement of water between compartments is intimately connected to the balance and movement of substances such as ions between the compartments. If the heart fails the levels of osmotically active compounds, such as plasma proteins, falls and so the osmotic potential of the blood decreases and swelling of the interstitial spaces, or oedema, occurs. Similarly, if the function of the lymphatic system is impaired then a process called lymphoedema can occur.

Questions

1   How is the molecular structure of water related to its function?
2   Explain the process of osmosis.
3   Compare and contrast diffusion, facilitated transport and active transport across plasma membranes.
4   How may oedema arise?
5   What part does the lymphatic system play in maintaining fluid balance between the blood and the interstitial compartment of the body?

Chapter 3

Body temperature regulation

Aim

To understand the regulation of body temperature.

Learning outcomes

This chapter will enable the reader to:

- explain what is meant by body temperature;
- describe and explain the source of body heat;
- recognise the importance of maintaining a constant body temperature;
- explain the mechanisms whereby body heat can be lost;
- explain the mechanisms whereby body heat can be conserved;
- recognise the implication any deviation in temperature control might have for patient well-being.

Introduction

The regulation of body temperature is another excellent example of a homeostatic mechanism that has already been referred to in Chapters 1 and 2. The human body is designed to work at a particular temperature and this temperature is maintained during health. If the temperature rises there are mechanisms for losing heat from the body and if the temperature falls there are mechanisms for generating and conserving heat in the body. However, as with all homeostatic mechanisms, they work within limits.

What is temperature?

Temperature is, strictly speaking, a measure of the movement of molecules. However, as the most common way to change the movement

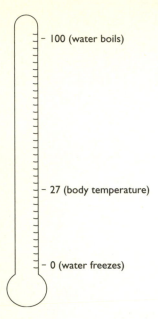

Figure 3.1 The centigrade scale for measuring temperature.

of molecules is by the application and removal of heat, we use temperature as a proxy measure for heat. Temperature is measured using the Kelvin scale and 0 Kelvin (−237 degrees centigrade) is referred to as absolute zero because, at this temperature, no molecular motion is possible. In other words, it is not possible to obtain a colder temperature than absolute zero. In everyday life, temperature is measured using arbitrary scales and in the United Kingdom and Europe the Celsius or Centigrade scale is used. This scale is zero at the temperature where water freezes (equivalent to 237 K) and 100 at the temperature where water boils (Figure 3.1). The normal body temperature, measured at the core of the body, is approximately 37 °C. Normal room temperature, for the purpose of scientific experiments, is usually 25 °C, just to give you some idea of what a temperature feels like, although most rooms are below this temperature and 25 °C actually feels quite comfortable.

Why do we need a constant body temperature?

Apart from water, the body contains inorganic and organic chemicals and the major organic component is composed of the biological molecules known as proteins. Proteins serve three functions in the body, they are nutrients, they form structures in the body such as skin and hair and they function as biological catalysts, facilitating and controlling the chemical reactions in the body. Proteins, which act in this last way, are called enzymes and their functioning is dependent on optimal body temperature.

Proteins are composed of long chains of amino acids and these chains conform in different ways. For example, keratin, the protein in skin and collagen, and in tendons and ligaments forms long chains. Other proteins, called globular proteins, fold up into specific shapes and more than one globular protein may be bound together. Enzymes are globular proteins and this makes them particularly sensitive to temperature. The shape of a globular protein is held together by many forces including strong covalent chemical bonds that are hard to disrupt. However, many of the forces, such as hydrogen bonds, are weak forces and these are susceptible, amongst other things such as pH and osmolarity, to changes in temperature. The function of an enzyme is dependent upon its shape and even small changes in shape can reduce its function. Therefore, the body strives to maintain a constant temperature in order to ensure the optimal function of the enzymes within it, which regulate everything from how we break down glucose to how well we repair a wound. Enzymes have optimum conditions under which they will work best and the optimum temperature for enzymes in the body is approximately 37 °C. If the body temperature falls below this the chemical reactions will slow down, as small changes in the shape of the enzymes will be induced thereby reducing their catalytic functions. If the body temperature rises, there will be an initial rise in the rate of chemical reactions – which is one of the purposes of a rise in our body temperature when we have an infection. However, if the temperature rises too much this will also induce changes in the shape of the enzyme and its catalytic activity will be reduced.

What is the source of body temperature?

Temperature is an indirect measure of heat and heat is a form of energy. Energy can be converted from one form into another and through the process of metabolism the body releases the chemical energy contained in the food we eat in order that it can be used in other chemical reactions, as mechanical energy by muscles and as heat. We are aware of the heat produced by the body when we take exercise, we become hot and take measures to lose heat from the body. However, even at rest, the body generates sufficient heat to maintain its core temperature and this is mainly achieved by the liver, which is a highly metabolically active organ, a major site of glucose breakdown and synthesis of other substances such as glycogen and proteins. Some tissues may exist solely to provide heat, a process known as thermogenesis, and brown adipose tissue may be such a tissue. Brown adipose tissue is more prominent in babies than in adults and this may be indicative of its function; small children lose heat very rapidly and are more susceptible to changes in body temperature generally. Brown adipose tissue synthesises and breaks down fat without any apparent product, other than heat, in a metabolic loop called a futile cycle but arguably very important in infants and small children.

Core temperature

When we talk about body temperature we are really referring to the core temperature of the body, in other words, the temperature in the core of the body – as opposed to the periphery – where the vital organs of the body such as the brain, the liver and the heart are located. Organs such as the liver produce heat continuously and, without some way of removing the heat from the core of the body, the core temperature would continually rise to a level where the enzymes in the vital organs would stop working. Clearly, this does not happen and this is due to the continual dissipation of heat from the core of the body to the periphery by the blood. In fact, one of the major functions of the circulation of blood is the transport and distribution of heat around the body.

Heat from the core of the body is transported around the body but, from the homeostatic perspective, it is the transport of heat to the surface of the body – the skin – which is most important as this is a means by which heat can be lost from the body. By controlling the extent to which heat is lost from the surface of the body, the extent to which heat is lost from or conserved by the core of the body is regulated. Once heat reaches the surface of the body it can be lost in a number of ways (Table 3.1): radiation – heat radiates from the body into the atmosphere provided that the atmosphere is at a lower temperature than the body, which is usually the case; convection – heat is convected away from the surface of the by the movement of air around the body; conduction – heat is conducted away from the body by contact with objects that are colder than the body; evaporation – body heat is used to evaporate water from the surface of the body. In the case of evaporation, the water on the surface of the body – provided, for example, by perspiration – changes from liquid water to water vapour without a change in

Table 3.1 Mechanisms of heat loss from the body

Mechanism	Characteristics
Radiation	The loss of heat directly to the atmosphere from the body.
Conduction	The loss of heat to colder objects with which the body is in contact.
Convection	The loss of heat to the atmosphere as a result of air currents passing over the body.
Evaporation	The loss of heat from the body in the conversion of water to water vapour on the surface of the body.

temperature and the energy for this change in state (i.e. from liquid to vapour) is provided by heat from the body. This heat is called the latent heat of evaporation because it is not detected by any change in temperature.

Loss of heat from the surface of the body is desirable in order to prevent the core of the body becoming overheated but there are circumstances under which we wish to increase the loss of heat from the surface of the body or to conserve heat and these are in addition to the homeostatic mechanisms to be described below – they are largely behavioural. For example, in order to increase heat conservation in the body we increase the environmental temperature in order to decrease the heat gradient from our bodies into the atmosphere, we put on more clothes in order to reduce the effect of convection and in order to insulate ourselves from colder objects. Conversely, if we want to lose heat from the body we will reduce the environmental temperature, remove clothing, generate drafts (e.g. using a fan) and we may even wet our bodies in order to increase evaporation from the surface of the body. In addition to the above behaviours, we may either curl up into a ball (e.g. in bed) when we are cold or spread out our limbs when we are warm and the objective here is to change the surface area of the body exposed to the environment: the larger the surface area exposed the greater the extent to which heat is lost.

Measuring temperature

Body temperature is measured using a thermometer: a device that measures temperature whether by the expansion of a liquid in a graduated tube, the relative movement of two metals in a bimetallic strip or one of the more sophisticated devices that uses a probe attached to an electronic device. When we measure body temperature we are trying to measure the core temperature and this is achieved by taking measurements in places where the core temperature is accessible but without having to invade the body. For these reasons temperature has traditionally been measured under the tongue, at the axilla (armpits), at the groin and rectally. At these sites major blood vessels pass close to the surface of the body and these will reflect the core temperature more closely than other sites on the surface of the body that are usually well below core temperature. The most modern method, now almost universal in the United Kingdom, is the use of tympanic membrane temperature, which is measured by inserting a probe, attached to an electronic meter, into the ear. This method has the advantages of providing a reading of core body temperature very quickly and it is as accurate as any of the other methods but suffers from few of their disadvantages. For example, measuring temperature orally can be influenced by hot and cold drinks, axillary temperature is inaccurate in very thin people because the thermometer does not come into contact with the skin and rectal thermometers are invasive. In the clinical setting, temperature measurement is commonly used along with pulse and blood pressure to monitor a patient's general condition and nurses are required to know how to carry this out correctly and knowledgeably, to record the results accurately and to report and respond to any deviations from normal such that the appropriate interventions are carried out.

The core temperature of the human body is 37 °C and a rise in temperature, called a pyrexia, often indicates that an infection is present. However, there are other causes of pyrexia. Conversely, a body temperature below 37 °C, or hypothermia, also indicates that something is wrong with the body. Pyrexia and hypothermia will be considered in more detail below after an explanation of how the body maintains, under most circumstances, a constant core temperature of 37 °C.

Temperature regulation

In addition to the behavioural aspects of temperature regulation described above, the body will regulate its own temperature, within limits, without any behavioural assistance. As mentioned above, this is achieved by altering the volume of blood reaching the surface of the body, the skin. The regulation of temperature is a homeostatic mechanism in which the detectors are the thermoreceptors in the skin

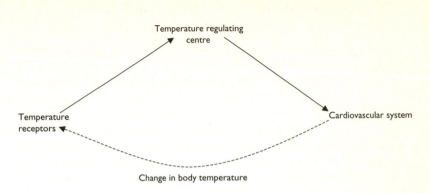

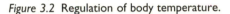

Figure 3.2 Regulation of body temperature.

(peripheral) and in the hypothalamus (central) (Figure 3.2). Both these sets of receptors provide information to the temperature regulating centre in the hypothalamus about body temperature, the peripheral receptors provide information about the environmental temperature and the temperature of the skin and the central receptors provide direct information about the core body temperature. Both these sets of information will trigger behavioural and homeostatic mechanisms. The control system for the regulation of body temperature is the hypothalamus, which will initiate homeostatic responses designed either to conserve or lose body heat and the effector system for the homeostasis of body temperature is the cardiovascular system, especially the capillary blood supply to the skin. Essentially, in response to a rising core temperature the temperature regulating centre initiates an increase in the blood supply to the skin, thus providing the 'flushed' look that the skin will adopt when it is warm. In response to a falling core temperature the temperature regulating centre initiates a decrease in the blood supply to the skin, which produces the pale appearance of skin when it is cold.

The system for temperature regulation involves negative feedback. If the core temperature is too high then the response is to promote heat loss from the body. Once the core temperature returns to normal then the mechanism for heat loss, the diversion of blood to the skin, is reduced. Conversely, if the core temperature falls then the response is to conserve heat by lowering the blood supply to the skin until the core temperature is restored to normal after which the blood supply to the skin is restored.

The mechanism of heat conservation and heat loss in the skin

The blood supply to the skin is composed of surface and deep blood vessels. When the body needs to conserve heat the blood flow to the superficial vessels is prevented and the blood flows to and from the skin via the deep blood vessels (Figure 3.3). When the body needs to lose heat the flow of blood is diverted to the surface vessels thus bringing heat to the surface of the body where it can be lost from the body by radiation, convection, conduction and evaporation. The flow of blood through either the deep or surface blood vessels is determined by precapillary sphincters, which are rings of smooth muscle in the blood vessels close to the capillary bed in the skin. When the body needs to lose heat the precapillary sphincters to the surface vessels are opened and those to the deep vessels are closed. There is an additional anatomical feature of the blood supply to the skin that maximises the blood flow to the surface and these are the arterial-venous anastomoses that connect the arterial and venous blood supply. The function of the anastomoses is to move blood directly from the arterial into the venous system without having to pass through the capillary system and this increases the blood flow to the surface. When the body needs to conserve heat the opposite situation prevails with the precapillary sphincters to the deep vessels open and the surface vessels closed. The opening and closing of the precapillary sphincters is controlled by the temperature regulating centre in the hypothalamus.

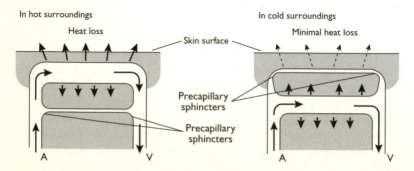

Figure 3.3 Diagrams to show heat loss and heat conservation from the skin surface: diagrammatic representations.

Counter-current exchange

Counter-current exchanges are common in nature. They are used in heat conservation mechanisms, in the function of the kidneys and in respiratory gas exchange. In terms of heat conservation and loss in the body, a counter-current system exists that is designed to conserve heat at the core of the body. As the arteries approach the surface of the body they are surrounded by a network of veins (vena comitantes), the purpose of which is to transfer heat from the arteries into the veins taking blood back to the core of the body (Figure 3.4). Heat will always move down a gradient from warmer to colder and the blood returning from the surface of the body has been cooled due to heat loss in the skin. When the body does not need to conserve heat, the shunting of blood to the

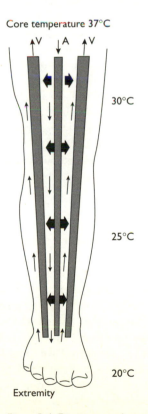

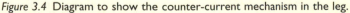

Figure 3.4 Diagram to show the counter-current mechanism in the leg.

surface vessels in the skin away from the deep vessels also serves the purpose of diverting blood away from the vena comitantes, thereby reducing heat conservation.

Perspiration

Bringing heat to the surface of the body is not, in itself, sufficient to ensure that heat is lost from the body. The four physical methods outlined above assist in this process and we can alter radiation, convection, conduction and evaporation behaviourally. However, there is also a physiological mechanism for increasing the amount of heat lost from the body by evaporation and this is the process of perspiration. There are glands in the skin called sudoriferous glands and these secrete sweat, mainly composed of water but also containing sodium and chloride ions, urea and other compounds onto the surface of the skin. The secretory activity is increased when the body core temperature is raised because the sudoriferous glands are controlled by the temperature regulating centre in the hypothalamus. When heat is brought to the surface of the skin it is used to evaporate the perspiration and heat is thus lost from the body because of the latent heat of vaporisation explained above. Clearly, when we produce more perspiration we lose water and salt from the body and, if we do not replace them, we are liable to become dehydrated. Therefore, there is a link here between two homeostatic systems; if we perspire and become dehydrated we will become thirsty and this will stimulate us to drink more. Dehydration will also initiate water conservation by the kidneys.

Generating heat

In addition to the behavioural strategies outlined above to conserve heat, we are also capable of deliberately generating heat in the body when we are cold and one of the major ways in which we do this is through muscle activity. It is not uncommon to see people moving their arms in order to generate heat but the best way in which to do this is to walk as we then exercise the largest muscles in the body, those of the upper legs through which a large volume of blood flows. The movement of large muscle means that energy sources are used and ATP is broken down to provide the energy for mechanical movement of the muscle. Such a process is not completely efficient and some of the energy released from ATP is lost as heat, which warms up the blood as it passes through the muscles and is transported to the core of the body. Paradoxically, this major method of heat generation can become a problem during heavy exercise, especially when the environmental temperature is high. Under these circumstances such heat generating activity runs alongside heat dissipating mechanisms. Thus, for example, the runner, whilst generating heat, will wear very light clothing and the body will be acting homeostatically to distribute blood away from the core of the body to the surface where it will be removed by convection and evaporation or perspiration.

In addition to the above mechanisms, which are voluntary, there is an involuntary mechanism called shivering whereby the body can generate heat from small but generalised and uncoordinated muscular contractions. The purpose behind shivering, which is controlled by the hypothalamus, is to increase the metabolic rate of the body, the rate at which it is using energy sources and thereby releasing heat energy from them. Shivering can double the metabolic rate very rapidly and is a short-term response to being cold.

In addition to shivering, which is a short-term response to cold exposure, the body can also slowly increase its metabolic rate over a few days in order to cope with movement to a cold environment or, alternatively, it can slow down the metabolic rate slowly in response to moving to a warm environment. These responses are also controlled by the hypothalamus but not directly through the nervous system. Rather, these responses are mediated hormonally and the hormones involved are the thyroid hormones, which are releases by the thyroid gland and controlled by the pituitary gland located on the base of the hypothalamus. Thyroid hormones have the effect, on metabolically active cells, of increasing their metabolic rate and this can contribute to the raising of the metabolic rate of the body. This slow metabolic response to changes in environmental temperature are the basis of acclimatisation. When people move from one climate to another and a significant change in temperature is involved they may take a few days in the new environment to adapt to the new temperature. During the process of adaptation, or acclimatisation, the hypothalamus is detecting that the environmental temperature has changed and, through its control of the pituitary, it is sending signals to the thyroid gland to produce and release more thyroid hormones into the blood or to produce less and release less. This explains why someone taking their holidays in a warmer climate may feel exhausted by the heat for a few days and, upon return to their usual colder climate, may feel cold for a few days until they re-acclimatise to their usual environmental temperature. It is generally the case that older people take longer to acclimatise than younger people and are more susceptible to the adverse effects of changing climates due to the fact that ageing decreases the ability of the hypothalamus to control metabolic rate through the pituitary and the thyroid glands.

Pyrexia and hyperthermia

Pyrexia is a normal response to invasion of the body by microorganisms and is part of the defence mechanisms against infection. The white blood cells that are active in responding to such invasion, of infection, release substances known as cytokines and interleukins, which are pyrogens that raise body temperature. The raised body temperature speeds up the enzymatic reactions and cellular processes associated with the non-specific and immune responses of the body. However, it should be noted that the actual cause of a pyrexia is not always known and that in older people it can be the case that infection is not always accompanied by pyrexia. While raised body temperature is beneficial to some extent, prolonged or increasing pyrexia leading to hyperthermia is potentially dangerous, and babies and small children are especially susceptible. The nervous system is particularly sensitive to hyperthermia and in adults this can lead to confusion, coma and even death – this is often called 'heat stroke'. Therefore, when people are showing signs of a marked pyrexia it is usual to take measures to try to reduce the body temperature back to normal. This can be achieved by enhancing the usual methods by which the body loses heat: clothing or bed clothing can be removed to increase radiation, tepid water can be applied to the body to increase evaporation, a fan can be used to increase convection but it should be noted that a fan aimed directly at the body or the use of cold water will cause peripheral vasoconstriction, which will be counter-productive as this will decrease heat loss from the surface of the body. However, it must be remembered that in pyrexia the core body temperature is rising because the hypothalamus is allowing it to. If you imagine the temperature regulating centre in the hypothalamus being like a thermostat that controls central heating in a house then, in pyrexia, the thermostat has been re-set to a higher temperature. Instead of 37°C, the thermostat will tolerate a higher core body temperature. The normal homeostatic corrective mechanisms will work but they will not work until the temperature has exceeded the normal core body temperature and reached a higher temperature. At the same time, due to this re-setting of the 'thermostat' a person with pyrexia will often feel that he/she is cold despite feeling warm to touch and having a higher than normal core body temperature. Unless the reason for the pyrexia is addressed either by removing infection from the body (antibiotics in the case of bacterial infections) or waiting until it has subsided (in the case of viruses) the body temperature will continue to be raised. On the other hand, it is possible to re-set the 'thermostat' in the hypothalamus using anti-pyretic drugs such as aspirin, paracetamol and ibuprofen. The precise action of these drugs is not known but they interfere with whatever aspect of infection acts on the temperature regulating centre in the hypothalamus and return the homeostatic mechanisms to regulate the core body temperature at 37 °C. The effect of these drugs is that the hypothalamus will now detect that the body core temperature is raised and will try to return the core body temperature to normal by enhancing the mechanisms for losing heat from the body. Primarily, blood will be directed to the periphery and perspiration will be increased and this is why when someone has a 'fever' and they take a proprietary medicine such as aspirin they are likely to perspire profusely and may report that they feel hot. It is often necessary to explain to patients that this is part of the mechanism of the body for losing heat and that they are not becoming warmer.

Hypothermia

Hypothermia is a condition in which the core temperature of the body falls below normal. However, clearly, there are degrees of hypothermia and it can range from mild discomfort to death. The usual cause is being exposed to a cold environment for too long and this can arise in extremely cold regions of the world such as the poles of the earth or at very high altitudes in mountainous areas of the world. It can also be caused by falling into the sea in temperate areas due to the speed with which the body loses heat when immersed in water. However, these are extreme cases and hypothermia can also occur in vulnerable individuals in cold weather at home and those most at risk are the very young and the very old but individuals with an underactive thyroid gland or advanced liver failure can also be at risk. Older people are at risk for a number of reasons and the primary one identified by community health care professionals is that they are more likely to be exposed to cold in the home due to low income and a determination to save money by using little heat in the home. This situation, which is essentially a social issue, is compounded by the fact that older people may be less able to detect that their body core temperature is low, they may not 'feel the cold' to the same extent. In addition, when they are cold the homeostatic mechanisms that help to protect the body against lowered core temperature will not be as effective in an older person.

As indicated above, there are degrees of hypothermia; in the initial stages the body will try to compensate through homeostatic processes but this ability will eventually be lost. The person with hypothermia will appear disoriented and weak initially in addition to having a low core body temperature. Ultimately, the person will become unconscious and at about 10 °C below normal body temperature the heart will stop beating and death will follow. Provided a person with hypothermia is found before the heart has stopped or significant brain damage has taken place it is possible to revive them by slowly rewarming the body. Ironically, the low core temperature will have slowed down the metabolic processes of the body and this may have a protective effect on vital organs. The body should not be rewarmed at more than about 1 °C per hour to avoid excessive vasodilation, heat loss and circulatory shock. In extreme cases, where no other course of action is possible, it may be necessary to place a person in a warm bath but the usual method of rewarming is to wrap in blankets, including space blankets that reflect heat back to the body, and to monitor closely the return of the body core temperature to normal.

Conclusion

The body strives to maintain a constant core temperature in order to ensure the optimal function of the vital organs that are contained there. Changes in temperature have a direct effect on the enzymes that control the metabolic activities of the body. In health, our first response to a change in temperature is behavioural but homeostatic mechanisms work to help the body to conserve or lose heat as appropriate. Heat homeostasis is achieved by the cardiovascular system, which alters the distribution of blood between the core and the surface of the body. Extremes of temperature are dangerous: hyperthermia and hypothermia can both lead to death and it is an important part of nursing care to monitor body temperature accurately and to take appropriate action to help the vulnerable person to regain a normal core body temperature.

Questions

1   Can you explain the relationship between temperature and heat?
2   How do changes in temperature outside of the normal range adversely affect the body?

3   With reference to the ways in which heat is lost from the body describe how each can be exploited in the loss and conservation of heat by the body.

4   How is negative feedback involved in the regulation of temperature?

5   In general terms, how does an antipyretic drug such as paracetamol work?

Chapter 4

Blood gases

Aim

To understand how the levels of oxygen and carbon dioxide in the blood are regulated.

Learning outcomes

This chapter will enable the reader to:

- explain why we have oxygen and carbon dioxide ions in the blood;
- describe how oxygen and carbon dioxide are transported in the blood;
- understand and describe the function of the respiratory system;
- understand and describe the control of the respiratory system;
- identify disorders that affect the blood gas levels;
- demonstrate knowledge of the precautions with oxygen therapy;
- understand the detrimental consequences of impaired blood gases on an individual's well-being.

Introduction

The blood gases are oxygen and carbon dioxide. Oxygen is required for metabolic processes such as the synthesis and breakdown of the biological molecules in the body and the release of energy from, for example, glucose, and for the storage of energy in high-energy compounds such as adenosine triphosphate (ATP). In the formation of ATP, oxygen combines with hydrogen atoms and forms water (Figure 4.1) and without this reaction the formation of ATP would not be possible. Oxygen is, therefore, essential for life.

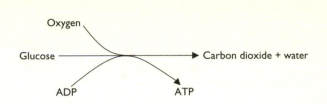

Figure 4.1 The involvement of oxygen in the production of ATP.

In the process of metabolism and the consumption of oxygen, the body produces carbon dioxide as this is produced at points in the metabolic processes when carbon atoms are removed from metabolic intermediate molecules, derived from, for example, glucose, and combine with oxygen. Carbon dioxide, therefore, is a waste product of metabolism and is removed from the sites where it is produced and, ultimately, removed from the body. The relationship between oxygen and carbon dioxide, therefore, may be crudely described by saying that oxygen drives the process of metabolism and carbon dioxide is the end product; an accumulation of excess carbon dioxide in the body will be harmful to metabolism.

The expression 'blood gases' refers to the levels of oxygen and carbon dioxide in the blood, which, in turn, is a proxy estimate of the extent to which the tissues of the body are receiving oxygen and removing carbon dioxide. In health, oxygen is constantly being supplied to the tissues and carbon dioxide and it is the measurement of blood gases that will primarily indicate whether the homeostatic mechanisms that regulate the levels of oxygen and carbon dioxide in the body are working within normal limits or whether, as in many disease states or disorders, there is a problem (Table 4.1).

Providing the tissues of the body with oxygen

Oxygen is a gas that constitutes about 16 per cent of the volume of the air we breathe and the body is able to remove oxygen from the air and transport it to the tissues and cells of the body. This process begins at the lungs, which are the two main organs occupying the greater part of the thoracic cavity (Figure 4.2). By increasing and decreasing the volume of the thoracic cavity (breathing) and thereby alternately decreasing and increasing the thoracic pressure, we are able to draw air into the lungs as we breathe in and to expel it as we breathe out. The air we breathe in

Table 4.1 Normal blood gas values

Substance	Partial pressure[a]
Oxygen	800–100 mgHg
Carbon dioxide	34–45 mmHg

Note
a   Blood gases are expressed in mm of mercury and
    as their contribution to the total pressure of gases
    (i.e. the partial pressure) in the blood.

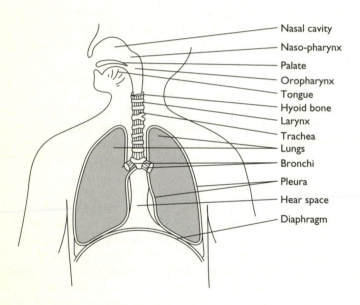

Nasal cavity
Naso-pharynx
Palate
Oropharynx
Tongue
Hyoid bone
Larynx
Trachea
Lungs
Bronchi
Pleura
Hear space
Diaphragm

Figure 4.2 Diagram of the respiratory tract.

(inspired air) is not the same as the air we breathe out (expired air): the inspired air has a higher content of oxygen than the expired air and the expired air has a higher content of carbon dioxide than the inspired air, which indicates, in part, the function of the lungs (Table 4.2). The lungs are responsible for providing the body with oxygen and for removing carbon dioxide from the body and this is achieved at the functional units of the lungs: the alveoli. The alveoli are microscopically small sacs at the end of the system of tubes that form the lungs and these sacs increase the internal surface area of the lungs to about the size of two tennis courts!

Table 4.2 Inspired and expired air compositions[a]

Inspired air (%)	
Oxygen	21
Carbon dioxide	0.03
Expired air (%)	
Oxygen	16
Carbon dioxide	4

Note
a The percentage of nitrogen is not shown.

Anatomically, the alveoli are intimately associated with the blood vessels through a system of capillaries that surround them, rather like a net bag. The purpose of the capillary network is to bring the blood into close proximity with the air in the lungs. The distance between the air in the lungs and the blood in the capillary network, the alveolar-capillary membrane, is microscopic and, because the interior of the lung is moist, the oxygen easily diffuses across the wall of the alveoli and the wall of the capillary into the blood. Following the same principle, carbon dioxide diffuses out of the blood and into the alveoli. The diffusion takes place because the concentration of oxygen in the alveoli is greater than the concentration of oxygen in the blood arriving at the alveoli and the converse is true for carbon dioxide (Figure 4.3). This explains why the composition of inspired and expired air differ: oxygen is being removed from the air in the alveoli and carbon dioxide is being produced. The fact that the lungs are being ventilated by the process of breathing means that the oxygen supply to the alveoli is being replenished when we breathe in while the carbon dioxide in the alveoli is being lost to the atmosphere when we breathe out.

Oxygen is not particularly soluble and only a few percent of the oxygen that crosses from the alveoli to the blood dissolves in the blood plasma – which is mainly composed of water. The majority of the oxygen enters the red blood cells that are packed full of the protein haemoglobin. Each haemoglobin molecule can bind four molecules of oxygen and where the oxygen concentration is high, as in the lungs, the binding between the haemoglobin and the oxygen is strong. On the other hand, where oxygen levels are low, in areas of the body that are metabolically active, the binding between the oxygen and the haemoglobin is weaker. The result of this variability in the strength of binding between oxygen and haemoglobin means that oxygen is taken away from the lungs in

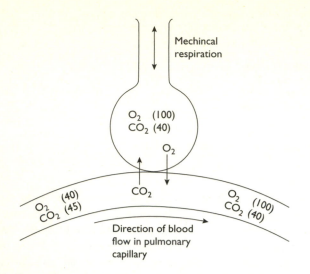

Figure 4.3 Gas exchange in the lungs. (All values in parentheses are in units of mmHg.)

the blood and then provided where it is needed. If the binding of haemoglobin to oxygen was the same in peripheral tissues as it is in the lungs then as red blood cells pass through the peripheral tissues, their oxygen content would remain intact and the peripheral tissues would not receive any oxygen.

In contrast to oxygen, carbon dioxide is more soluble and dissolves in the plasma to a greater extent. However, most of the carbon dioxide is also carried in the red blood cells because, once dissolved, carbon dioxide enters red blood cells where it is converted with water by an enzyme called carbonic anhydrase into carbonic acid (Figure 4.4). This is then broken down into bicarbonate ion and hydrogen ion thereby effectively lowering the level of carbon dioxide. A concentration gradient of carbon dioxide is set up across the red blood cell membranes. The concentration of carbon dioxide is higher outside the cell in areas of the body where carbon dioxide is being produced (e.g. muscles) and higher inside the cell where carbon dioxide is being removed (the lungs). As a result, carbon dioxide diffuses into the red blood cells in the peripheral tissues and diffuses out of the red blood cells at the lungs because the chemical reactions described above are reversible: the hydrogen ion and the bicarbonate ion can combine to produce carbonic acid, which is broken down by

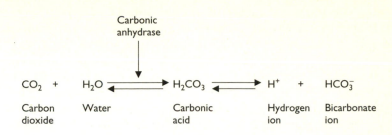

Figure 4.4 The reaction catalysed by carbonic anhydrase.

carbonic anhydrase into carbon dioxide and water. This reverse reaction is important in helping the body to get rid of excess acid (hydrogen ions) from the blood as will be explained below.

Homeostasis and blood gases

The demand for oxygen by the body and the production of carbon dioxide is not constant. When we are going about our normal daily lives we require more oxygen and produce more carbon dioxide than when we are resting and this situation is made even more acute by exercise where the demand for oxygen by the muscles increases and the production of carbon dioxide also increases over our normal daily levels. However, despite this, the body manages to maintain relatively constant levels of blood gases and this is another excellent example of homeostasis involving a detector, an effector, a control centre and negative feedback. The consequences of not maintaining blood gases within certain limits would be detrimental to the body. If the oxygen levels in the blood fell then there would be insufficient oxygen to provide for the metabolic activities of the tissues and this must be maintained whether the body is at rest or working hard. A failure of sufficient oxygen to meet cellular metabolic demands is essentially what is meant by the term shock. Conversely, if the levels of carbon dioxide in the blood became too high then it would no longer be possible to remove carbon dioxide from the metabolically active tissues because the concentration gradient that drives the process of carbon dioxide diffusion into red blood cells in the peripheral tissues would be lost.

Contrary to popular belief, it is the changing levels of carbon dioxide in the blood and not the levels of oxygen that is the primary stimulus for the homeostatic control of blood gas levels. This control is achieved through the respiratory system (the effector) with the respiratory centres in the hypothalamus as the control centre and specialised nerve endings at specific locations in the cardiovascular system and the central nervous system, called chemoreceptors, which are the detectors of carbon dioxide levels in the blood (Figure 4.5). Oxygen levels have to be very low before they have any significant influence on respiration. This is probably due both to the fact that the supply of oxygen to the blood is very high and, more particularly, the fact that the haemoglobin in the red blood cells in arterial blood is usually almost 100 per cent saturated with oxygen within a normal range of activity. In other words, oxygen levels in the blood are not particularly sensitive to changing circumstances. On the other hand, the changing levels of carbon dioxide in the blood will be a very early and sensitive indicator of changing circumstances, such as the beginning of exercise. Furthermore, the respiratory system is 'driven' by carbon dioxide levels in the blood. If we hyperventilate – breathe in and out very quickly – we will maintain blood oxygen levels but will, relatively quickly, deplete blood carbon dioxide levels and this is detrimental. We will feel light headed and experience tingling in our fingers and toes and may even lose consciousness – which is the body's way of forcing us to breathe normally. If someone is hyperventilating, something that can happen in anxiety attacks, then re-breathing the air they are exhaling, preferably using a paper bag, will increase the levels of carbon dioxide they are inhaling and, in turn, the levels of carbon dioxide in the blood and a normal rate of breathing will be restored.

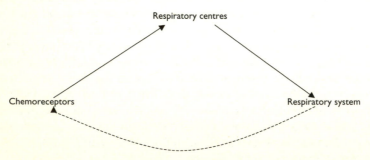

Respiratory centres

Chemoreceptors

Respiratory system

Change in blood gas levels

Figure 4.5 Regulation of blood gas levels.

There are two types of chemoreceptors. The peripheral chemoreceptors are located in the carotid sinus and in the aortic arch and the central chemoreceptors are located in the medulla oblongata of the brain. The peripheral chemoreceptors are strategically located in order to monitor the carbon dioxide levels of the blood as it leaves the heart and also as it enters the head to supply the brain. The central chemoreceptors, which do not come into direct contact with the blood, monitor the levels of carbon dioxide in the cerebro-spinal fluid (CSF) that bathes the brain – clearly another strategic monitor of the carbon dioxide levels as an increase in carbon dioxide levels in the CSF could endanger the metabolic activity of the brain. The central chemoreceptors respond to changing levels of hydrogen ion because the carbon dioxide in the CSF dissolves and carbonic anhydrase, the enzyme that was present in red blood cells and is ubiquitous in the body, leads, as has been said, to the production of hydrogen ions. The peripheral chemoreceptors respond to the changing blood levels of carbon dioxide and hydrogen ion and also to changing levels of oxygen.

The chemoreceptors provide information on carbon dioxide levels to the respiratory centre in the medulla of the brain. Essentially, an increase in carbon dioxide levels stimulates respiration and the increase in respiration serves the purpose of providing the blood with more oxygen and removing carbon dioxide more rapidly from the blood due to increased ventilation. While both the rate and depth of respiration are increased it is mainly through increased depth of breathing – moving greater volumes of air in and out of the lungs with each breath – that greater ventilation takes place. If you take exercise such as running you will notice that, while you are exercising, your rate of breathing will not be much greater than normal although when you stop it may well increase. This is possibly concerned with repaying the 'oxygen debt' that occurs in the body after exercise has ceased. Once the carbon dioxide levels in the blood have returned to within normal limits, negative feedback will reduce the stimulus to the respiratory centre and the rate and depth of respiration will be reduced as a result.

The respiratory system also plays a part in the homeostasis of acid/base balance in the body, which is worth mentioning in the present context because the mechanism is shared with the one described above for regulating carbon dioxide levels in the blood. The acid/base balance in the blood is measured in pH units, which are a measure of the hydrogen ion concentration. Hydrogen ions are produced as a by-product of metabolic reactions and too many (or, indeed, too few) is detrimental to the body as vital body enzymes operate at optimal pH levels – analogous to the optimal temperature range referred to in Chapter 3. If the hydrogen ion concentration increases then the pH becomes lower and the body tries to maintain a neutral pH (approximately pH 7.4) in the blood. As described above, the peripheral chemoreceptors can respond directly to hydrogen ion concentration and the result of this stimulus is the same as rising carbon dioxide levels – in fact, carbon dioxide and hydrogen ion levels will often rise simultaneously. The respiratory system will be stimulated in terms of rate and depth and more carbon dioxide will be removed from the blood to the atmosphere at the lungs as a result of the increased ventilation. The acidity of the blood is reduced because the enzyme carbonic anhydrase breaks carbonic acid down into carbon dioxide and water. This removal of carbonic acid leads to the removal of hydrogen ions as they are then combined with bicarbonate ion to replace the carbonic acid that has been removed.

Alterations in blood gas levels

Homeostatic mechanisms for maintaining blood gas levels will, like all homeostatic mechanisms, only work within a certain range. Beyond this range the body will suffer from altered blood gas levels: usually raised levels of carbon dioxide and lowered levels of oxygen and this can range from being debilitating to being life-threatening. A range of disorders will lead to alteration in blood gas, which can result from reduced lung function or from reduced capacity of the blood to carry oxygen.

Lung function can be reduced in many ways such as by the restriction of entry and exhalation of air to and from the lungs (as in asthma and bronchitis), by an increase effectively in the distance the gases have to diffuse between the alveoli and the blood due to the accumulation of fluid in the lungs (as in pneumonia or pulmonary oedema) or by a decrease in the ability of the lungs to expand and recoil after breathing, called compliance (as in emphysema). Each of these conditions will result in a decreased delivery of oxygen to the blood and a decreased delivery of carbon dioxide to the alveoli.

The cardinal sign that a person has a respiratory problem such as any of those above is that they will suffer from shortness of breath (dyspnoea). A person with lung disease such as bronchitis or emphysema may purse their lips as they exhale in an effort to maintain air pressure in the lungs and prevent the collapse of the airways in order to maximise the benefit from each breath.

A person who has difficulty with breathing may find that a change in position will help them to breathe more easily and should be helped to sit in whatever position is comfortable and beneficial. Sitting up will relieve the pressure on the respiratory diaphragm from visceral organs, which push against the respiratory diaphragm while lying down. However, sitting up may not be the best position for breathing from the perspective of blood gases because, when a person is sitting up, gravity will act on the blood in the lungs such that the lower portions of the lungs may be well perfused while the upper portions of the lungs are poorly perfused. Some people find that sitting up and leaning forward gives them the greatest relief from their dyspnoea.

If the lungs are working to optimal capacity then the blood gases can be altered by factors in the blood that affect, adversely, the capacity of the blood to carry oxygen. These conditions include the various types of anaemia in which the amount of haemoglobin in the blood is reduced either through a reduction in the amount of circulating red blood cells, as would occur in acute blood loss, or due to a reduced level of haemoglobin of the right quality in the red blood cells. This may be due to dietary factors such as iron deficiency or due to chronic bleeding as may occur with peptic ulcers. However, the capacity of the blood to carry carbon dioxide will not be altered. The person with anaemia, other than that caused by a massive bleed, will suffer from very vague symptoms initially such as tiredness, headaches and dizziness without any very specific symptoms. However, if the anaemia progresses, the capacity of the blood to carry oxygen will diminish to such an extent that the person will experience shortness of breath and the oxygen deficit will be detectable in blood gas analysis. An interesting phenomenon occurs in people with anaemia, that is, their blood contains higher than normal levels of a substance (2,3-diphosphoglycerate) that makes the haemoglobin more likely to give up its oxygen at lower oxygen concentrations in the blood and this may be an adaptive mechanism to encourage the provision of oxygen to peripheral tissues.

Finally, another condition in which the capacity of the blood to carry oxygen is affected is carbon monoxide poisoning. Carbon monoxide binds to haemoglobin molecules in such a way as to prevent, essentially irreversibly, the binding of oxygen and this can happen at very low concentrations of carbon monoxide. At first carbon monoxide poisoning has no symptoms but, by the time the person with carbon monoxide poisoning detects symptoms, such as tiredness and dizziness, and the late signs of a cherry pink skin, it may be too late and, indeed, may be fatal.

The effect of low oxygen levels in the blood is that the peripheral tissues become poorly supplied with oxygen, they become hypoxic. The outward signs that someone is hypoxic may include cyanosis, a bluish discolouration of the peripheral aspects of the body, especially the lips and the mucous membranes. People who are hypoxic for long periods, such as those with chronic respiratory disease, for example, chronic bronchitis, may display a sign called 'clubbing' whereby the ends of the fingers become enlarged and assume a 'clubbed' appearance. The reasons for clubbing are not understood but result from engorgement with blood vessels at the ends of the fingers and may be an effort to ensure adequate blood circulation to the peripheral tissues of the body.

Oxygen therapy

Oxygen therapy is an obvious adjunct to any condition where a person is short of breath. However, it is more likely to be effective for conditions where the lungs are failing to provide adequate oxygen to the blood than in conditions where the blood has reduced oxygen carrying capacity. In the latter case, no matter how much oxygen you deliver to the blood, it will only be able to carry what its haemoglobin content will allow it to carry once all the haemoglobin is saturated. As an example, it used to be common for athletes to be given oxygen after a race. However, this practice has ceased as it serves no purpose. At the end of a race an athlete, whose lungs will be healthy, will be ventilating the lungs to their maximum and supplying the blood with large amounts of oxygen: the haemoglobin in the athlete's blood will be fully saturated and the provision of additional oxygen via the lungs will not increase the oxygen levels in the blood.

However, where the lungs are failing to provide adequate oxygen to the blood, oxygen therapy must be administered with caution. Oxygen, except in emergencies, should only be given when prescribed and the diagnosis of the person and any other medication being taken have been taken into account. Oxygen, in prolonged high concentrations, is actually a very toxic substance to the body, a fact all too well appreciated in the mechanically ventilated patient. We survive in an oxygen-poor environment; oxygen is only present in the air we breathe at approximately 16 per cent of the volume. Furthermore, in some conditions, such as chronic bronchitis, the administration of oxygen in too high a concentration can be fatal. The chemoreceptors of people with chronic respiratory disease, due to the chronically high levels of carbon dioxide in the blood (hypercapnia), lose their sensitivity to carbon dioxide levels in the blood and depend, instead, on hypoxia to drive respiration. A sudden increase in the level of oxygen in the blood will, effectively, switch off the hypoxic respiratory drive. As a result, a patient with any form of chronic obstructive airways disease will require, alongside optimal positioning, controlled oxygen therapy. In all patients having oxygen therapy of any sort it should always be remembered that oxygen is highly combustible and appropriate precautions in this respect taken.

Conclusion

Oxygen drives the metabolism of the body and carbon dioxide is the waste product. Both gases co-exist in the blood and the relative levels in the blood are an indicator of the functioning of the respiratory system. The respiratory system functions to exchange oxygen and carbon dioxide between the blood and the atmosphere; it is also responsive, through homeostatic mechanisms, to the changing conditions of the body in terms of the demand for oxygen. It is, however, except in people with chronic respiratory conditions, the levels of carbon dioxide in the blood that regulate the respiratory system.

Questions

1   Can you explain how oxygen and carbon dioxide are exchanged between the lungs and the atmosphere?
2   How are oxygen and carbon dioxide transported in the blood?
3   Explain the part negative feedback plays in the regulation of respiration.
4   In what ways may the level of oxygen in the blood be adversely affected?
5   Why is it necessary to take precautions with oxygen therapy?

Chapter 5

Blood pressure

Aim

To understand the purpose and regulation of blood pressure.

Learning outcomes

This chapter will enable the reader to:

- understand how blood pressure is created;
- explain the function of blood pressure;
- describe the components of blood pressure;
- explain negative feedback and blood pressure control;
- demonstrate what is meant by high blood pressure and low blood pressure;
- understand the implication of abnormal blood pressure for an individual;
- understand what is meant by heart failure and its consequences.

Introduction

Most people are familiar with the structure of the heart and with its role as a pump within the cardiovascular system. Moreover, most people are familiar with the general concept of blood pressure in terms, particularly, of the adverse effects of high blood pressure. The aim of this chapter is to explain the origin and purpose of blood pressure and how the homeostasis of this important physiological phenomenon is maintained. We have already encountered the concept of pressure within the cardiovascular system in Chapter 2, where we saw that hydrostatic pressure played a role in the exchange of fluids between compartments of the body. In fact, hydrostatic pressure is exactly the same as blood pressure; osmotic pressure is not relevant in the large blood vessels because they are impermeable to water. It is only in the capillary beds, between the end of the arterial system and the start of the venous system, where the blood vessels are permeable to water, that osmotic pressure and hydrostatic pressure exert a combined effect of the exchange of fluids between the plasma and the other fluid compartments of the body (see Figure 2.3).

The origin or source of blood pressure is the pumping action of the heart as it pumps blood into a limited volume: the cardiovascular system. The blood pressure, therefore, is a function of the volume of blood being ejected from the heart, the cardiac output, and the degree of difficulty with which that blood fills the blood vessels it is entering – this is called resistance. In the case of the cardiovascular system, the resistance is referred to as peripheral resistance as the central blood vessels, those close to the heart, have very large diameters and, therefore, offer very little resistance. The resistance in the cardiovascular system is provided by peripheral blood vessels, the arterioles, as will be explained below.

The stroke volume is a function of the rate at which the heart is beating and the volume of blood ejected from the heart with every beat. The volume of blood in the healthy body remains constant but the heart rate can change in order to accommodate different circumstances and demands upon the cardiovascular system. The peripheral resistance can also be changed by varying the diameter of peripheral blood vessels and we will return to the part that these vasoactive mechanisms play in regulating blood pressure below. Varying the diameter of blood vessels is normally the only way in which the blood pressure is varied. It should be noted, nevertheless, in a fluid system, that the pressure in the system can be varied by varying the viscosity of the fluid in the system or by varying the length of the system. However, the length of the cardiovascular system remains constant and, except in extreme cases of dehydration, the viscosity of the blood remains constant and, therefore, these factors play no part in the control of blood pressure.

Measuring blood pressure

Blood pressure is normally measured in the arteries and the usual site of measurement for clinical purposes is in the brachial artery in the arm, which is at the point where the arm bends at the opposite side from the elbow, where the brachial artery runs quite close to the surface. Figure 5.1 shows the common sites on the body where pulses may be felt.

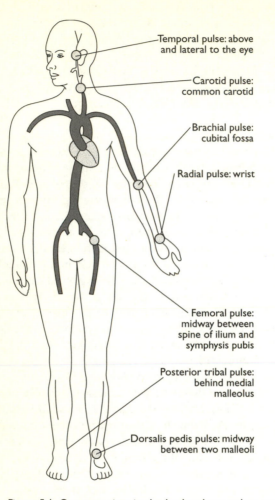

Temporal pulse: above
and lateral to the eye

Carotid pulse:
common carotid

Brachial pulse:
cubital fossa

Radial pulse: wrist

Femoral pulse:
midway between
spine of ilium and
symphysis pubis

Posterior tribal pulse:
behind medial
malleolus

Dorsalis pedis pulse: midway
between two malleoli

Figure 5.1 Common sites in the body where pulses can be felt.

Blood pressure is expressed in terms of the systolic and diastolic blood pressures (i.e. systolic/diastolic) and measured in millimetres of mercury (mmHG). This measurement of blood pressure is an indirect measurement requiring a sphygmomanometer, a cuff and stethoscope. The cuff consists of an inflatable cloth-covered bladder and is connected to an inflation–deflation bulb via a control valve. Tubing attaches the cuff to the sphygmomanometer (Figure 5.2). The brachial artery is

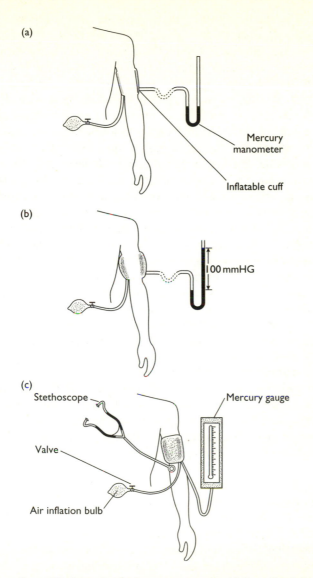

(a)

Mercury
manometer

Inflatable cuff

(b)

100 mmHG

(c)

Stethoscope

Mercury gauge

Valve

Air inflation bulb

Figure 5.2 Principle of sphygmomanometry: (a) the cuff is deflated; there is no pressure in the cuff, and the mercury levels in the two arms of the U-tube manometer are the same (in actual clinical sphygmomanometers mercury is stored in a reservoir and not in a U-tube as shown here); (b) the cuff is inflated; pressure in the cuff is equal to the difference in height between the two mercury levels; (c) the auscultatory method for measuring systolic and diastolic pressures.

located by palpation and the cuff (of the appropriate size) is applied to the patient's arm 2–3 cm above the antecubital fossa with the centre of the cuff bladder over the artery. The cuff is then inflated to a pressure greater than the systolic pressure in the artery. (The systolic pressure can be initially estimated by palpating either the radial or brachial pulse and inflating the cuff until the pulse disappears). Although more sophisticated electronic devices are available for the continuous monitoring of blood pressure, when using the mercury sphygmomanometer, the blood pressure can be recorded by the application of the head of the stethoscope over the brachial artery and the cuff slowly deflated at a rate of 2–3 mmHg per second. As the cuff is deflated, and the artery begins to open, pulsating or tapping sounds are heard (called Korotkoff sounds) and when these begin is taken to indicate the systolic blood pressure, that is, the blood pressure when the heart is contracted. The sounds continue changing in quality as the artery progressively opens. The point at which the sounds become muffled or disappear is taken to indicate the diastolic blood pressure, that is, the blood pressure when the heart is relaxed. The origin of the Korotkoff sounds is not fully understood but the appearance of these sounds could be a result of the blood starting to pulse through the brachial artery when the pressure in the cuff falls below the systolic pressure. Possibly the sounds continue as long as some pressure, above the diastolic pressure, is being applied to the cuff and when the pressure falls below the diastolic the sounds disappear.

There is no such thing as a 'normal' blood pressure but, in a healthy adult, a blood pressure of 120/80 mmHg would be considered normal. The effect of disease and age on blood pressure will be considered below but, generally speaking, it is changes in the diastolic pressure that are of most concern as an indicator of disease and disorder affecting the blood pressure.

Some expertise is required in the measurement of blood pressure as measurements between individuals and between times by individuals can be different. It is important that the person is relaxed, that (after the initial measurement in both arms) the same arm – usually the left arm – is used each time and that the appropriate size of cuff is used for the size of the patient's arm. Otherwise, unless lying and standing blood pressure is being specifically recorded, the patient should be seated and the spyhygmomanometer should be positioned level with the heart. The arm should be relaxed and supported and so positioned that the cuff is also at heart level.

The systolic and diastolic blood pressures can be used to estimate other important aspects of blood pressure such as the pulse pressure, which is the difference between the systolic and diastolic blood pressures. In the case of a normal health adult with a blood pressure of 120/80 mmHg, the pulse pressure is 40 mmHg. If the diastolic blood pressure were to rise to 100 mmHg then the pulse pressure would drop to 20 mmHg. The pulse pressure is affected by three factors: the amount of blood pumped with each beat (the stroke volume), the speed at which the blood is ejected and the distensibility of the arteries. In arteriosclerosis, for example, where the arteries become stiff, the pulse pressure is chronically raised. Equally, in significant blood loss or dehydration, the pulse pressure will fall.

Another expression of blood pressure is the mean arterial pressure (MAP), which gives the average pressure driving the blood into the tissue throughout the cardiac cycle. MAP is expressed as a third of the difference between the systolic and diastolic blood pressures plus the diastolic pressure. Thus, a person with blood pressure of 120/80 mmHg would have a MAP of about 93 mmHg. It is expressed in this way because diastole lasts slightly longer than systole and the importance of MAP is that it is the blood pressure which fills the coronary arteries which supply the heart muscle with blood. Clearly, it can be crucial to know the MAP, especially in critical care situations. This can be seen when we consider the coronary arteries, which unlike the rest of the cardiovascular system, are not being supplied with blood during systole. Due to the contraction of the heart muscle these arteries become occluded and only fill with blood during diastole and the pressure that provides the coronary circulation is the MAP.

Why do we have blood pressure?

There is, perhaps, a lay perception that 'blood pressure' is a bad thing which is derived from the fact that abnormally high blood pressure is harmful to health. However, blood pressure within normal limits is a very good thing; indeed, we could not survive for very long without it. Witness the effects of a very sharp decline in blood pressure: at the very least we faint but there can be more serious and even life-threatening consequences.

The blood has several functions but all of these are dependent upon the supply of blood to tissues being continually replenished and removed and this is only achieved by the effective circulation of the blood. This applies equally to the supply of nutrients to tissues with the removal of waste products as it does to the distribution of heat around the body. While most are familiar with the pumping action of the heart – as mentioned above – the role of pressure in the circulation of blood is less well appreciated. In fact, the heart exists to produce the pressure within the cardiovascular system and it is the gradient of pressure: high to low, between the left ventricle of the heart to the right atrium of the heart that is the reason for the circulation of the blood. The blood is ejected from the left ventricle of the heart under very high pressure; nowhere else in the cardiovascular system is blood pressure as high. The major blood vessels close to the heart, such as the aorta, are elastic in order to absorb the changes in pressure that they undergo between the relaxation (diastole) and the contraction (systole) of the heart. The elasticity of these blood vessels, which include the brachial arteries and the renal arteries, generally speaking, direct blood towards the major organs of the body such as the lungs and the kidneys, they play no part in the control of blood pressure – their function is to direct blood away from the heart as quickly as possible, under pressure, to the major organs of the body. After the elastic arteries there are muscular arteries, the diameter of which, under the control of the autonomic nervous system, can be varied due to the concentric rings of smooth muscle in their walls. By varying the diameter of these blood vessels the blood can be directed towards tissues where it is required and restricted from other tissues in order to accommodate this. The blood in the muscular arteries remains under high pressure but not as high as in the elastic arteries. After the muscular arteries the blood is delivered to the capillary beds in the tissues by the arterioles that are small in diameter and this is where the resistance to blood flow in the cardiovascular system occurs. In particular, this is where, when the heart is at rest, diastolic pressure is maintained. In addition, it is through varying the diameter of the arterioles that blood pressure is controlled.

The blood from the arterioles, which is under high pressure, enters the capillary beds of the tissues where, despite the reciprocal relationship between diameter and pressure, the blood pressure drops to a few mmHg due to the combined diameter of the capillaries in the tissues which is much greater than the diameter of the arterioles entering the tissues. The drop in pressure means that the blood flow through the capillaries is sufficiently slow for the exchange of oxygen, carbon dioxide, nutrients and waste products of metabolism to take place.

As the blood leaves the capillary beds it is gathered up into the venules, which have a smaller diameter than the combined diameter of the capillary bed, and the blood pressure rises slightly. The blood is returned to the heart via the venules, which take blood to the veins and major veins, such as the venae cavae. However, the blood pressure in the veins is insufficient, on its own, to return blood to the heart and the venous system is designed to assist the process of blood circulation. For example, the veins of the lower limbs run between deep and superficial layers of skeletal muscle and there are valves that prevent the blood from flowing down the limb. The blood is directed up the limbs, through the valves, by the action of the muscles: as they contract, the blood is 'milked' up the veins. This system is called the skeletal muscle pump and its importance can be witnessed in people who have to stand still for prolonged periods, especially when it is hot, such as soldiers on parade. It is not uncommon for people to collapse under these circumstances because insufficient blood is being returned to the heart from the lower limbs and, thereby, the blood supply to the brain is reduced with an obvious and dramatic effect. Collapsing to the horizontal position actually serves to restore the blood circulation.

Under the circumstances described above, people can be given the advice to wiggle their toes thereby operating the skeletal muscle pump in the legs. A similar system is thought to operate in the thorax with the alternating pressures that take place as we breathe in and out: as we breathe out and reduce the pressure in the thorax, blood moves into the lungs and is prevented from being expelled when we breathe out by venous valves analogous to those in the legs.

Control of blood pressure

Blood pressure has to be maintained within reasonable limits to ensure, on the one hand, a constant circulation of blood. On the other hand, a very high blood pressure is harmful in several ways, as will be discussed below, and the blood pressure, therefore, should not be allowed to rise so high as to damage the body. The mechanism for controlling blood pressure has all the components of a classic homeostatic system incorporating negative feedback (Figure 5.3). The control centres for the blood pressure is in the brain, specifically in the medulla – where other control centres that we have discussed are also situated. The detectors for blood pressure are the baroreceptors (baro = pressure), which are located throughout the cardiovascular system but especially in the aortic arch and the carotid sinuses where they are co-located with the chemoreceptors. There are also baroreceptors in the venous sinus where blood returns to the right atrium from the upper and lower regions of the body. The effector for the homeostatic control of blood pressure is the cardiovascular system, which responds via changes in the heart rate and in the diameter of the arterioles.

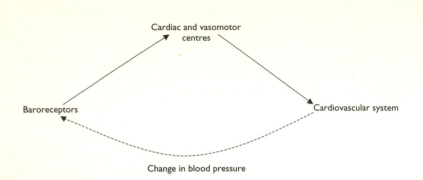

Figure 5.3 Regulation of blood pressure.

The control of blood pressure is exerted via changes in heart rate and blood vessel diameter because blood pressure is a function of cardiac output and peripheral resistance. Blood pressure will be altered either by a change in cardiac output, which in itself is a function of the heart rate and stroke volume, or by altering the diameter of the arterioles and thereby peripheral resistance. The arterioles are always slightly constricted at rest due to the constant stimulation of the sympathetic nervous system, and this phenomenon is called vasomotor tone.

The baroreceptors are designed to detect stretch in the blood vessels where they are located and this stretching is transmitted as nerve signals to the medulla where the signals can be interpreted and acted upon by the cardiac centres. The location of the baroreceptors is strategic in the sense that the aortic arch will be the first location in the body to detect the pressure of the blood as it is ejected from the heart. The baroreceptors in the venous sinus will detect the blood pressure in the venous system at the point where blood is being returned to the heart. The baroreceptors in the carotid sinuses detect blood pressure in the blood that is supplying the brain. The brain is very sensitive to changes in blood pressure both in terms of low blood pressure leading to poor blood supply and possible collapse. Equally, the blood vessels in the brain are very sensitive to high blood pressure and may rupture with dramatic and fatal results. The rupture of a blood vessel in the brain is referred to as a cerebrovascular accident, commonly referred to as haemorrhagic 'stroke'. The baroreceptors in the atrial sinus also detect an increase in blood pressure in the venous system and send signals to the cardiac centres in the hypothalamus to lower blood pressure.

The baroreceptors detect changes in blood pressure, if the blood pressure increases then the blood vessels become stretched and signals are sent to the cardiac centres in the medulla. Stimulation of the baroreceptors by an increase in blood pressure has the effect of slowing down the heart rate, on the one hand, and causing vasodilatation on the other. The cardiac centre concerned with accelerating the heart rate is inhibited and the cardiac centre concerned with slowing the heart rate is stimulated leading to slowing of the heart. The vasomotor centre, which maintains cardiovascular tone, is inhibited leading to vasodilatation. The slowing of the heart rate reduces the cardiac output and the vasodilatation decreases the peripheral resistance and both of these actions lead to a reduction in blood pressure. As described above, the mechanism of regulating blood pressure involves negative feedback: once the blood pressure has been returned to within normal limits then the stimulation of the baroreceptors ceases and the inhibitory effect on the cardiac accelerating centre and the vasomotor centre ceases and the stimulation of the cardiac inhibitory centre also ceases.

In the case of a fall in blood pressure the converse set of circumstances applies: the baroreceptors detect the fall in blood pressure and the signals they send to the medulla become inhibited leading to the cardiac accelerating centre being stimulated and the cardiac inhibiting centre being inhibited and this leads to acceleration of the heart. At the same time, the vasomotor centre is stimulated leading to vasoconstriction and an increase in peripheral resistance. The combination of increased heart rate and increased peripheral resistance leads to an increase in blood pressure. Once the blood pressure is restored to within normal limits, the baroreceptor stimulation will be initiated and the effects on the cardiac and vasomotor centres leading to increased blood pressure will cease. This is another example of negative feedback. When blood pressure falls the chemoreceptors, which play a part in the control of respiration as explained in Chapter 4, also play a role. A drop in blood pressure, which has the consequence of reducing the blood supply to the tissues thereby reducing oxygen levels and increasing carbon dioxide levels in the blood, is detected by the chemoreceptors. The chemoreceptors also send signals to the cardiac centres and the vasomotor centre and have the same effect as the inhibition of the baroreceptors by reduced blood pressure.

Clearly, in the control of blood pressure, as we go about our daily lives, the demands on the cardiovascular system are constantly changing. For example, standing up from a sitting position puts an instant demand on the cardiovascular system to ensure that the brain receives enough blood: standing up means that the effects of gravity on the blood in the body will be increased and there will also be an increased demand for blood by the legs. The baroreceptors in the carotid sinus will detect a fall in blood pressure and in order to ensure that the blood supply to the brain is not decreased there will be an increase in vasomotor tone and heart rate compared with the sitting position. Some people who cannot readily make this homeostatic adjustment to standing up may faint or feel giddy and suffer from a condition known as postural hypotension. This is more common among older people and is a demonstration of the reduced homeostatic ability, which is a feature of ageing. In fact, most people will experience a giddy sensation on occasions when they stand up too quickly – especially if they have been sitting or sleeping for a long time. These effects will be exacerbated by such things as alcohol and being in over warm surroundings such as a hot bath; both alcohol and being over warm will cause generalised peripheral vasodilatation, which reduces the blood pressure and also means that less blood is available centrally to be diverted to the brain with the change in posture. The effect of a sudden, significant and prolonged fall in blood pressure (hypotension), whereby there is inadequate perfusion of body tissues, characterises shock, considered in Chapter 8.

The constantly changing demands upon the body mean that, in common with other homeostatic systems, the apparent 'steady state' of blood pressure within normal limits in the body is, in fact, achieved by a balance between the effects of signals from the baroreceptors on the cardiac and vasomotor centres.

Hypertension

The term hypertension means raised blood pressure but when this is used as a clinical description it means that the blood pressure is abnormally and persistently raised. However, a precise definition of what constitutes hypertension is not easy and age must be taken into account as both the systolic and the diastolic blood pressures tend to rise with age. As an example, a 20-year-old person with a blood pressure of 140/90 mmHg may be considered to be hypertensive but not a 75-year-old person in whom a blood pressure of 170/105 mmHg might be considered abnormal.

Blood pressure is essential to the circulation of the blood but clinical hypertension is potentially damaging to the body. Abnormally high blood pressure may lead to the rupture of the delicate blood vessels in the brain with devastating consequences as mentioned above. In the blood vessels hypertension causes thickening in the tunica media (the middle layer of a blood vessel) and accelerates the development of atherosclerosis and increases peripheral resistance. This results in an extra strain on cardiac functioning in that the heart must necessarily work much harder to eject blood. Hypertension may also damage the delicate mechanism of glomerular filtration in the nephrons of the kidney leading to renal failure. Hypertension is a cause of great concern not only for its obvious consequences on the equilibrium of the body's functions but also because in the early stage, the abnormality is without symptom and the pathology may only be detected by chance, for example, at a routine examination for some other reason. If hypertension is prolonged then it will ultimately lead to heart failure. Initially, the heart will increase in size to accommodate this extra workload, just like a skeletal muscle will with exercise. However, unlike skeletal muscle, the heart has no opportunity to rest completely and the heart will eventually become damaged and begin to fail. The consequences of heart failure were covered previously but will be summarised below as the problems of heart failure are, essentially, problems of blood pressure in the venous system.

Heart failure and blood pressure

Heart failure is a failure of the heart to fulfil its normal function of pumping blood into the cardiovascular system to ensure optimal tissue perfusion. When the heart fails the main problem is not one of insufficient blood supply to peripheral tissues, or to the lungs. Problems initially arise because blood in the venous system is not cleared leading to an increase in venous blood pressure there and, thereby, hydrostatic pressure leading to problems that will be explained below.

The heart has two sides with the right-hand side of the heart collecting blood from the venous system and circulating it to the lungs, where it becomes oxygenated, and the left-hand side collecting blood from the lungs and circulating it around the rest of the body. Clearly, the consequences of right- and left-sided heart failure will be different and we will consider right-sided heart failure, which is more common, first.

Right-sided heart failure may arise for a variety of reasons including such things as atrial fibrillation and chronic obstructive airways disease. When the right side of the heart fails this will create a backlog of blood in the venous system and the blood pressure here will rise, which will have consequences in the capillary beds. The consequences of this process were described in Chapter 2 and will only briefly be described here. In the capillary beds an exchange of fluid is possible between the blood and the surrounding tissues because the capillaries are permeable to water – unlike the remainder of the cardiovascular system. The exchange of fluid is under the influence of the blood pressure, or hydrostatic pressure, inside the capillary and the osmotic pressure inside the capillary: the hydrostatic pressure tends to push fluid out of the capillary and the osmotic pressure tends to draw fluid into the capillary. At the arterial end of the capillary bed the hydrostatic pressure exceeds the osmotic pressure and fluid is pushed out of the capillaries and into the surrounding tissues. By so doing the hydrostatic pressure falls and at the venous end of the capillary system the osmotic pressure exceeds the hydrostatic pressure such that fluid is drawn back into the capillaries. Any excess fluid pushed out into the peripheral tissues is removed by the lymphatic system that returns fluid to the cardiovascular system at the subclavian veins.

Under normal circumstances, therefore, there is no excessive build up of tissue fluid. However, if the right-hand side of the heart fails the hydrostatic pressure will increase at the venous end of the capillary bed and may even exceed the osmotic pressure here with the consequence that excessive tissue fluid occurs. This fluid is under the influence of gravity and will accumulate at the points in the body which are lowest. Therefore, the cardinal sign of right-sided heart failure is accumulation of fluid in the peripheries of the body leading to swelling. If someone is sitting or standing, fluid will accumulate in the ankles leading to swelling, which is called oedema. This type of oedema is known as pitting oedema: if the swollen area is pressed lightly with the fingers then pits will be formed. Left-sided heart failure commonly results from such disorders as coronary artery disease and, of course, hypertension. The consequences of failure of the left side of the heart lead to increased blood pressure in the pulmonary veins that clear blood from the heart to the left ventricle. The effect of an increase in this system is that fluid is forced out of the pulmonary circulation and, as there is no interstitial space in the lungs, into the alveoli leading to the phenomenon of pulmonary oedema. The accumulating fluid impairs respiration and causes coughing up of pink frothy sputum; frothy because the fluid is mixed with air and pink because it contains red blood cells that have been pushed from the capillaries. Unresolved pulmonary oedema may lead to symptoms of right-sided heart failure through a backlog of pressure from the left side of the heart, through to the right side of the heart.

Conclusion

Blood pressure is essential to the circulation of the blood. The pumping action of the heart and the constriction of the peripheral blood vessels contributes to blood pressure and, through homeostatic mechanisms including negative feedback, variations in these parameters is used to regulate blood pressure. Blood pressure can be too low, hypotension, which leads to poor perfusion of peripheral tissues, or to high, hypertension, which has many adverse effects on the body. If the heart fails to pump efficiently then the main consequence is a build up of pressure in the venous system leading to peripheral oedema, in the case of right-sided heart failure, or pulmonary oedema, in the case of left-sided heart failure.

Questions

1   What is the relationship between cardiac output, peripheral resistance and blood pressure?
2   Explain how blood pressure can be measured.
3   How does blood pressure ensure the circulation of the blood?
4   Describe how blood pressure is regulated by negative feedback.
5   What may lead to increased venous pressure and what might the consequences be?

Chapter 6

Repairing damage

Aim

To understand the mechanisms whereby the body repairs damage and deals with invasion by microorganisms.

Learning outcomes

This chapter should enable the reader to:

- understand and describe haemostasis;
- describe the processes in blood clotting;
- understand what is meant by clotting disorders;
- describe the process and explain the purpose of inflammation;
- explain non-specific and 'specific' immunity;
- understand and describe the principles of wound healing.

Introduction

The book thus far has covered a series of homeostatic mechanisms that constantly make corrections in the conditions when the body is experiencing change. For example, the changing demands on the cardiovascular system, as we undertake exercise in terms of increasing blood pressure to cope with the increased need for circulating blood and the need to maintain a constant body temperature have been considered. The parameters within which the above mechanisms work can be considered to be 'normal' and if the body experiences circumstances outside of the parameters within which the above mechanisms work this could be considered to be 'abnormal'. The mechanisms to be described in this chapter share one property with the homeostatic mechanisms previously described in the sense that they attempt to return the conditions of the body to normal. Nevertheless, these mechanisms have their limits and will not cope with infinite deviation from the body's normal status.

This chapter will, however, consider a set of responses of the body that are stimulated, usually, through injury. The particular set of responses described here ensure that the body does not lose too much blood, can respond to infection and can repair any damage to the skin. Specifically, this chapter will cover haemostasis, inflammation and wound healing. The initiation of the cellular mechanisms that fight infection will also be considered.

Injury

The kind of injury we will be concerned with in this chapter is quite minor and one from which the body would be expected to recover. As such we will consider minor cuts and grazes rather than major trauma from which the body is unlikely to recover without significant medical assistance. Such injuries will penetrate the protective layer of the skin and the blood vessels immediately below the surface of the skin – the capillaries. Such an injury presents the body with three immediate challenges: to stop the bleeding that occurs as a result of damage to the blood vessels, the repair of the broken skin and the prevention of infection to the body. If loss of blood is not prevented then continual bleeding will eventually lead to a significant reduction in the volume of the circulation and this potentially will precipitate shock (to be addressed in Chapter 8). If the skin is not repaired then the body is vulnerable to dehydration and infection. If infection goes unchallenged then the tissues of the body will be invaded by microorganisms (bacteria, viruses and fungi) and these will eventually lead to a toxic condition with possibly devastating consequences.

Haemostasis

Haemostasis is the process whereby bleeding is stopped and it consists of four processes: blood vessel constriction, formation of a plug, formation of a blood clot and contraction of the clot.

The four phases of haemostasis identified above are an integral part of the wound healing process and are, collectively, known as the vascular phase of wound healing. Each phase will be described below.

The first phase of haemostasis, occurring within seconds of injury, involves spasm in the muscular layer of the blood vessels. This serves to reduce the diameter of the damaged blood vessels thereby reducing blood flow in the area and reducing blood loss. This effect can last for up to 30 min and it is worth knowing about as it can save lives, even in cases of severe injury to arteries. When an artery is severed, the blood is under high pressure and will spurt out under the influence of the pumping action of the heart. If you encounter someone with an arterial bleed the appropriate first aid is to apply firm pressure to the area where the bleeding is taking place. The reduction in the blood flow, due to the pressure, will allow the vascular spasm in the artery to reduce the bleeding to a steady flow. The bleeding should then be sufficiently reduced to allow you to take further first aid action such as summoning help, moving the injured person away from further danger, or the danger away from the injured person and, if appropriate, placing the patient into the recovery position. You may then be able to improvise a dressing for the wound, which can be applied firmly and held in place by adhesive tape or by using an improvised bandage until a proper dressing can be obtained.

The formation of a plug takes place when one of the cellular components of blood, the platelets, come into contact with the damaged blood vessels. This causes them to swell and change shape and, in the process, they become sticky and adhere to each other and to the fibres of a protein found in skin called collagen, which have been exposed at the site of injury. The adhered platelets release substances that act as chemical messengers (thromboxanes) and these encourage the activation of more platelets that arrive at the site of injury, change shape and adhere to the platelets already there, and to the collagen, forming a plug at the site of injury and this prevents further blood loss. At the same time as the platelets are arriving and adhering the blood clotting process has already begun and this adds strength to the plug.

Blood clotting, or coagulation, is very complex and the purpose of this process is to produce a filamentous protein called fibrin, which forms a mesh-like network of fibres at the site of injury. The fibrin mesh strengthens the plug and leads to the cessation of bleeding. Fibrin is an insoluble protein that is made from a soluble protein called fibrinogen. This conversion from a soluble to an insoluble form of this protein is necessary because, if the insoluble form were present in the blood then it would lead to damage by the premature occlusion of blood vessels and this would lead to the cessation of blood flow to vital areas of the body, especially parts of the brain or the heart.

The response of blood vessels to injury, however, is to activate the processes whereby fibrin is made and these processes can be summarised as beginning with the synthesis and release into the blood of the enzyme thrombokinase (also known as thromboplastin) from damaged cells. The events triggered by this enzyme, in turn, lead to conversion of another protein, prothrombin, into an enzyme called thrombin and it is thrombin that is directly responsible for the conversion of fibrinogen into fibrin (Figure 6.1).

There are two pathways whereby thrombin is produced and these are known as the extrinsic and intrinsic pathways. The extrinsic pathway is activated directly by the tissue damage and leads quite directly and quickly to the production of thrombin more or less as described above. The effect of the extrinsic pathway lasts only for a few minutes.

The intrinsic pathway is stimulated by damage to the epithelium of the blood vessels and causes the platelets to aggregate and burst, releasing chemical factors that initiate the intrinsic pathway. The intrinsic pathway works by what is known as a cascade mechanism, whereby each step in the pathway stimulates the next step meaning that a relatively small stimulus due to blood vessel damage at the beginning of the cascade leads to a large response at the end of the cascade thereby amplifying the initial stimulus. The effect of the intrinsic pathway takes a few minutes to produce thrombin but this effect lasts for about 30 min. The result of the two pathways working together means that there is a rapid response to

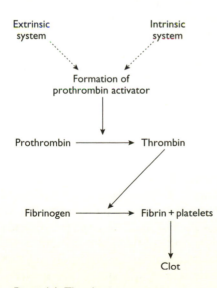

Figure 6.1 The clotting process.

injury, in terms of thrombin production, followed by a longer acting effect that is large enough to lead to adequate haemostasis. The end result of both pathways, therefore, is the same: the production of thrombin that leads to the formation of insoluble fibrin.

A large number of factors is involved in the clotting mechanism, more so in the intrinsic than the extrinsic pathway. Calcium is a requirement of both pathways. If any of these clotting factors is missing in the blood, usually the result of inherited genetic disorders, then the clotting mechanism will be impaired. In the intrinsic pathway lack of certain factors (VIII, IX and XI) lead to disorders collectively known as the haemophilias. Lack of factor X leads to a similar disorder. In the absence of these factors, blood clotting is significantly impaired and severe bleeding may occur either spontaneously or from very minor injuries. Consequently, life for a person with haemophilia may be restricted by the fact that they have to be very careful in their daily lives not to sustain even minor injuries such as those that may result from sporting activities. However, should bleeding episodes occur the absent factors can be isolated from blood donations and administered by intravenous infusion. Although not without its side-effects, by so doing, the individual is enabled to lead a reasonably normal life.

A milder disorder of haemostasis occurs in people with a lower than normal number of platelets in their blood and this is known as thrombocytopaenia. This condition results in superficial bleeding and bruising and may only result in significant loss of blood following surgery or extraction of a tooth. The causes of thrombocytopaenia include autoimmune conditions where the immune system of the body fails to recognise some of its own components, in this case platelets, and attacks and destroys them. Equally, disorders of the bone marrow or taking some medicines, for example, certain anticancer drugs, can also lead to a reduction in platelet numbers.

On the other hand, there are disorders of the haemostatic system that lead to an increased tendency for blood to coagulate, which is potentially damaging to health, as mentioned above. Such disorders arise out of a combination of factors such as the deposition of fatty deposits on the inner surface of arteries, changes in the behaviour of platelets and changes in blood clotting factors. Any single abnormal blood clotting event is likely to be any combination of these. Deposits on the walls of arteries lead to turbulence and slowing of the flow of the blood, which increases its tendency to coagulate, and if this is combined with changes in the clotting system then the chances of a clot occurring are increased. It is possible that small clots are regularly formed and reabsorbed in the blood but it is the size and site of clots that will lead to damage to the body and any abnormalities in the clotting system will increase the likelihood of larger clots. A clot in the blood circulating to the brain may lead to a cerebrovascular accident; in the heart to a myocardial infarction and in the lungs to a pulmonary embolus. Each of these events may be fatal and each, at least, will inflict damage upon the organs of the body where they occur due to occlusion of blood vessels and, thereby, a marked reduction in the supply of oxygen to the tissues supplied by the vessels where the clot has occurred.

A particular type of clotting disorder that has gained media prominence in recent years is deep vein thrombosis due to its association with, the so called, 'long haul' flying. This usually takes place in the deep veins of the legs and is a result of venous stasis, or blood pooling in the lower limbs. We considered the mechanisms for the return of blood from the lower limbs in earlier chapters and saw that this mechanism, involving the venous valves, was dependent upon movement in the lower limbs, which is required in order to compress the veins and move the blood in the direction of the heart. Deep vein thrombosis is a risk for people who are immobilised for long periods – as in 'long haul' flying – or in patients who are recovering from surgery, especially orthopaedic surgery, whose limbs may have been immobilised. A deep vein thrombosis is a painful event but the real danger of a deep vein thrombosis is that small clots can break off from the main clot in the lower leg and become lodged in the coronary or pulmonary blood vessels where a myocardial infarction or a pulmonary embolus could follow, which could lead to death.

The best approach to the problem of deep vein thrombosis is clearly to prevent thrombus formation in the first place. This can be achieved by ensuring that the muscles of the leg are kept active. This is best accomplished by wiggling the toes in order to keep the skeletal muscle pump working or, provided that you are not immobilised, by getting up and walking around every hour. In addition, it is advisable to drink plenty of fluids (non-alcoholic) as dehydration may contribute to the development of deep vein thrombosis. Patients who are immobilised can be advised to wiggle their toes and if they are unable to do this then anti-embolic stocking may be worn. These elasticated stockings provide graduated compression increasing blood flow in the deep veins and preventing the pooling of blood in the lower limbs.

In the event that someone is unfortunate enough to suffer a thrombosis then there are a number of approaches to treatment, all of which can be understood on the basis of the clotting mechanism described above.

These approaches include parenteral (i.e. introduced by injection as opposed to swallowed) anticoagulants, oral anticoagulants and thrombolytic drugs that are introduced by intravenous injection. The most common anticoagulants are heparin (parenteral) and warfarin (oral) and both of these are used following a thrombosis in order to discourage the formation of further blood clots. Anticoagulants are also used to prevent the formation of thrombosis, for example, prior to heart valve surgery, which will cause turbulence at the site of the valve and thereby increase the risk of clotting.

Heparin, given intravenously or subcutaneously, acts by blocking several of the steps in the blood clotting mechanism by antagonising (i.e. preventing the action of) several of the factors involved in the intrinsic pathway of blood clotting. Warfarin, given orally, antagonises the action of vitamin K, which is essential for the synthesis of several of the factors involved in the intrinsic pathway for blood clotting. Clearly, the use of anticoagulants is not without risk and the risks can be considerable if the dosages of the anticoagulants and their subsequent effect on the clotting mechanisms are not monitored closely. Reducing the efficiency of the clotting mechanism leaves the person who is receiving anticoagulant therapy prone to severe bleeding from even minor injuries.

Sensible advice to men on anticoagulant therapy, for example, is to stop shaving with a wet razor and both men and women should use a soft toothbrush. Otherwise, they must be vigilant about the signs of excessive abnormal bleeding such as haematuria (blood in the urine) and spontaneous bruising. In addition to taking precautions, there are laboratory tests that are performed on samples of blood from the person undergoing – or about to undergo – anticoagulant therapy. The details of such tests, such as the prothrombin time and the international normalised ratio that are used in patients using heparin and warfarin, respectively, are beyond the scope of the present volume. However, generally speaking, they investigate how long it takes for a sample of blood, from a person having anticoagulant therapy, to clot compared with either a control or a standard. If the time taken for the blood to clot is excessive then it indicates that the dosage of the anticoagulant should be reduced. In addition to the anticoagulant substances above, there is a class of substances called thrombolytic agents and these are enzymes that are capable of digesting blood clots. Thrombolytic agents are now routinely administered following a myocardial infarction and are effective in saving lives. There are specific contraindications to the use of these drugs and their use, increasing the risk of bleeding, requires close monitoring.

Antiplatelet drugs differ from anticoagulant drugs and they are used to prevent the aggregation of platelets, which lead to thrombi. Aspirin, a drug used for many years as an analgesic and antinflammatory agent, is an effective antiplatelet drug and is used in low daily doses to reduce the risk of strokes and myocardial infarction in vulnerable people. Recently, other antiplatelet drugs such as clopidogrel and ticlopidine have been introduced.

Inflammation

Inflammation is a protective response of the body to injury and a response that serves the purpose of providing a non-specific, as opposed to the specific response by the immune system, to the invasion of the body by harmful cells, pathogens such as bacteria and viruses. Inflammation is also important in stimulating the process of wound healing, which will be considered in the next section.

The most obvious sign that inflammation has taken place after injury is that the area that is injured becomes reddened, warm, swollen and painful. Despite the discomfort for the injured person, it is important to realise that inflammation is a necessary part of the response of the body to injury.

Injury to tissues causes the localised release of substances that increase the blood flow to the area and the leakage of fluid from the blood into the tissues. The substances released include histamine, which is responsible for the discomfort and discolouration that accompanies inflammation. These substances increase the permeability of the blood vessels in the injured area and this leads to the swelling. The increased localised pressure in the area due to the accumulation of tissue fluid also leads to localised pain because of increased pressure on the nerve endings (nociceptors) around the injured area.

The increased permeability of the blood vessels allows white blood cells called macrophages and neutrophils to leave the blood and enter the tissue spaces. These cells are phagocytic cells, which means that they can surround, ingest and digest any harmful cells such as bacteria and viruses. Other blood-borne protein substances known as complements may be activated to amplify the inflammatory and immune responses needed to destroy pathogens. This process is described as being non-specific because it takes place regardless of the type of pathogen that is present and ingests them regardless. However, this non-specific process is essential in stimulating the specific response of the body to such invasion and is better known as immunity. Immunity is specific because it enables the body to mount a response via cells called lymphocytes, which respond to particular types of bacteria and viruses that enter the body. This, in turn, enables the body to mount a generalised response to any particular type of pathogen that may enter the body and thereby the blood and infect other parts of the body. Moreover, the immune response also has 'memory' because the body can 'remember' invasion by any particular type of harmful cell and mount a more rapid and effective response if this type of cell invades the body again. The immune response is mediated by the lymphocytes that respond by producing cells (T lymphocytes) that specifically ingest harmful cells and cells (B lymphocytes) that produce specific proteins called antibodies, which attach to harmful cells destroying and inactivating their toxins. These harmful cells are known also as antigens, the term derived from its ability to generate an antibody reaction.

The link between the non-specific and specific responses is made by the phagocytes that are also described as antigen presenting cells (APCs). Once they have digested the harmful cells, these APCs combine parts of the antigens with proteins called major histocompatability proteins. These are moved to the plasma membranes of the phagocytes where they are, thereby, presented to the immune system and stimulate the production of the specific lymphocytes and the memory cells. This quite complex process enables the body to respond rapidly and more effectively following a subsequent invasion.

Wound healing

Wound healing is the process whereby breaks in the continuity of the skin – caused either by injury or by the planned trauma of surgery – are repaired in order to restore the integrity of the skin and, thereby, its protective functions. The processes of haemostasis and inflammation are part of the process, and necessary precursors to the two final stages of wound healing. The product of haemostasis (fibrin) is essential to wound healing and the process of inflammation, which, as described above, is essential for the non-specific and immune reactions to injury, is also essential to the process of wound healing.

Before considering the process of wound healing in more detail it is worth noting that, from the perspective of wound healing, there are two types of wound. Some wounds merely involve regeneration of the epidermis while others are deeper, requiring repair of the deeper layers of the skin and regeneration of the blood supply to the skin. In the superficial wound the epithelial cells migrate over the wound surface while in deeper wounds – of which surgical wounds are an excellent example – the underlying layers have to be repaired in advance of the epidermis being replaced. In order that all the stages are covered here we will consider the healing of a deep wound (Figure 6.2).

Inflammation is often considered to be the first stage of wound healing. The process of proliferation that follows consists of granulation, contraction and epithelialisation. Granulation is the result of angiogenesis, the production of new blood vessels, in the deep wound. At the same time as the new blood vessels are developing, the macrophages, which have been brought to the site of injury by inflammation, stimulate the production of fibroblast cells and these use the fibrin fibres laid down during haemostasis in order to migrate into the wound and begin producing ground substance and collagen fibres.

Following granulation the fibroblasts produce contractile proteins that pull the edges of the wound together, reducing the wound size: the contraction phase of wound healing. Finally, in the proliferation phase, new epithelium grows back over the wound and this epithelium either migrates in from the edge of the wound or arises from hair follicles that have been left intact in superficial wounds. The epithelium stops

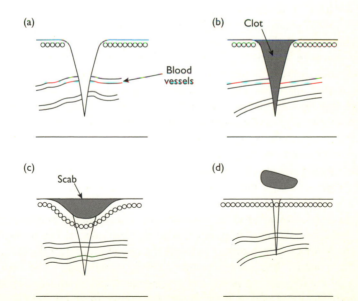

Figure 6.2 Wound healing: (a) Injury; (b) Clotting; (c) Migration, granulation, proliferation; (d) Maturation.

growing over the wound once the wound is fully covered – presumably when the new cells come into contact with one another. If there is a scab present from blood that has coagulated on a wound then the epithelium grows underneath the scab which is then removed from the wound. In minor wounds it can still take several days for the process from injury to removal of the scab to take place.

When the above processes are complete the process of maturation of the wound begins. This can take varying lengths of time according to the severity of the wound. For major wounds the process may take as long as 2 years. Maturation involves the strengthening of wound by the collagen fibres, the removal of any blood clot by destruction of the clot – described above – and the reduction of blood supply to the wound until it contracts and flattens leaving an area of the skin in which hair follicles and sweat glands do not regenerate.

Nursing and wound care

Nurses have the prime responsibility for the care of wounds and their care of wounds must be based on an understanding of the processes of haemostasis, inflammation and wound healing described above. A great many factors influence the healing of wounds such as the age of the person with the wound, their nutritional status, whether or not they smoke, have any comorbidity (associated conditions, e.g. diabetes mellitus, which may influence the course of wound healing) or whether they are taking medication, principally corticosteroids, which may impair wound healing.

However, apart from elective surgery, people usually do not choose to have or prepare for having a wound and, therefore, will present following minor injury, trauma and emergency surgery before which there has been no opportunity to address any of the issues that may influence the process of wound healing. Therefore, nurses are usually presented with the cleansing and dressing of wounds and it is their participation in this which can influence the course of healing. There is considerable evidence to support the use of occlusive, moist and warm environments for the healing of wounds and the majority of products on the wound dressing market are designed to promote such an environment. The occlusive nature of dressings is required to lower the oxygen levels on the surface of the wound – but not to exclude oxygen completely – and this is thought to stimulate the process of angiogenesis and granulation of the wound. The moist environment is also conducive to granulation and is essential for epithelialisation of the wound following granulation. It is also considered unnecessary to sterilise the wound by using antiseptic fluids. Some of these are directly harmful to the wound and, in any case, complete sterility may reduce the inflammatory response by removing pathogens and thereby reducing the necessity for macrophage cells at the site of injury, which are an essential part of the process as they stimulate the production of fibroblasts. In order to cleanse wounds the use of normal saline or water is recommended – even tap water in certain wounds is recommended as opposed to sterile water. Vigorous swabbing of the delicate wound surface must also be avoided as this may cause damage and cleansing, if required, should be by irrigation. If a wound does become infected then it is better to have antibiotics prescribed than to change the regime of wound management. If necrotic (dead) material is present in the wound then it needs to be removed either by effective irrigation pressure or by using a special topical application. In established necrotic wounds where hard, dry devitalised eschar is present, this may need to be removed surgically.

The issue of how often to change a wound dressing is not easy to answer except by saying 'as often as required'. One of the main factors in making a decision will be the integrity of the dressing that is in place. If the dressing becomes damaged, is leaking excessively round the edges or striking through the dressing, then this can lead to infection. This may be an indicator to change the dressing but, especially in a recent surgically induced wound, it may be better to cover the original dressing with a larger dressing as this will avoid disturbing the wound, reducing the moisture levels at the surface of the wound and allowing the wound to cool down. All of these will slow the wound healing process, especially in the early stages. Clearly, excessive and continued bleeding from the wound needs to be investigated, for example, a surgical wound may require to be surgically repaired. Some of the wound dressing materials available are transparent films and these have the advantage of allowing the nurse to observe the wound without removing the dressing. Nurses should be aware that a wound in which white fluid (pus) has accumulated and which is visible through such a dressing is not an indication that the wound is infected nor that the dressing needs to be removed and changed. This accumulation of white cells is a normal part of the wound healing process and is a necessary stimulant for the healing process: removing the dressing and cleaning the wound will have an adverse effect.

Conclusion

The body is periodically subject to injury and invasion by microorganisms. Injury can lead to bleeding and breaks in the continuity of the skin and the body has specific mechanisms to deal with bleeding and wound healing. The process of inflammation is crucial to both the process of wound healing and protection from invasion by microorganisms through non-specific and specific immunity. Nurses need to understand the processes of inflammation and wound healing in order to provide appropriate care. Wound management is very much the domain of nursing care and nurses can do a great deal to enhance the homeostatic goals of wound healing.

Questions

1   How does the body protect itself from excessive bleeding?
2   How can the blood clotting process become disordered?
3   What advice would you give someone taking anticoagulant therapy?
4   Explain how inflammation is a valuable process.
5   What is the link between non-specific and specific immunity?
6   Describe the stages of wound healing.
7   How can nurses facilitate wound healing?

Chapter 7

Cancer

Aim

To understand the nature of cancer from a homeostatic perspective.

Learning outcomes

This chapter will enable the reader to:

- understand the nature of cancer;
- understand and describe how cancer can develop;
- describe and explain how cancer may spread;
- identify the causes of, and risk factors associated with, cancer;
- identify how the risk of cancer might be avoided or minimised;
- describe the different approaches to the treatment of cancer.

Introduction

The subject of cancer may seem like a radical departure from the material contained in the book up to this point, which has mainly been concerned with the natural functioning of selected systems of the body. Cancer is different as it concerns, potentially, all of the systems of the body and is, in a sense, the antithesis of homeostasis. However, cancer has consequences for homeostasis in the body and, in fact, arises from a deviation from homeostasis of one process that begins soon after fertilisation of a human ovum by a sperm cell and continues until we die: the process of cell division. Studying cancer lets us see how a loss of homeostasis in one particular system, even in only one part of the body, can have devastating consequences for the rest of the body and may even lead to death. On the other hand, an understanding of cancer, its development and consequences, also equips nurses to accompany patients with cancer through what is called 'the cancer trajectory', which increasingly ends in successful treatment for an increasing range of cancers. It will also help nurses to explain the nature of cancer to patients, why they may have it and what can be done for them and the important fact that not all cancers are the same. On the other hand, some cancers do inevitably lead to death and this is one aspect of nursing where nursing care comes to the fore in terms of helping patients towards a peaceful death and through all of the potential pain, discomfort and distress that they may face. Much of this care is based on an understanding of many of the aspects of homeostasis that have been covered up to this point in the book.

What is cancer?

Cancer is a proliferation of abnormal cells in the body and these cells are referred to as neoplasms because they represent new growth. The somatic cells (as opposed to gametes) divide by a process called mitosis whereby the genetic material in the cell is normally doubled and distributed equally between the two new cells prior to division. This process is continually repeated in order to replenish the tissues and, thereby, the organs of the body. Some tissues require to be replaced rapidly, such as the tissue lining the mouth and gastrointestinal tract because it is constantly exposed to friction, as food is chewed, swallowed and digested. In other rapidly growing parts of the body such as the skin, cells are also rapidly dividing but in other organs such as the brain the rate of division is slower. Whatever the rate of cell division, it is appropriate for the tissues and organs in question and it stops when there are sufficient cells. In other words, it is under homeostatic control: it is accelerated by growth factors when new cells are required and slowed down when there are sufficient new cells. A perfect example of this process was provided in Chapter 6 in relation to normal wound healing. When the skin is wounded, the epithelial cells divide and migrate across the surface of the wound. However, once the surface of the wound is covered then the cells stop dividing. In homeostatic terms, there is a negative feedback mechanism working whereby the stimulus to produce new cells is turned off.

In the case of cancer, the homeostatic mechanisms related to cell division fail and abnormal cells, derived from the tissues in which they are located, divide in an uncontrolled manner. Such cells are not dependent on the presence of growth factors to simulate their growth and division and they are not subject to the usual mechanisms that stop cell growth and division when there are sufficient new cells. Collections of cancer cells in tissues can be palpable or visible by X-ray – for example, cancer of the prostate gland or the lung – and such a collection of cancer cells will be called a tumour. However, cancer may also be evident in the absence of a tumour, for example, in leukaemia where there is a proliferation of abnormal blood cells.

How does cancer arise?

Cancer is, essentially, a disease arising as a result of mutation in the genetic material of our cells. Our genes contain deoxyribonucleic acid (DNA), which provides a code for all the activities of a cell: the proteins it makes, the substances it takes into the cell and those it excretes and the rate at which the cell grows and divides (Figure 7.1). The double helical structure of DNA is familiar to most people and this aspect of DNA explains how it is able to reproduce prior to cell division and conserve the genetic code. The genetic code contained in sections of DNA arises from the unique sequences of sub-units (bases) in specific parts of DNA molecules. This sequence of bases is used to code for a template molecule called RNA and this is used, in turn, as a template for the synthesis of proteins, which are the molecules that allow cells to carry out all their activities. If anything goes wrong with the coding sequence in DNA this is referred to as a mutation. Mutations arise constantly at a very low rate and it is reckoned that no two cells in any tissue are identical. Mostly, the body can tolerate such a low level of mutation in its DNA and there are mechanisms working within cells to correct them. Therefore, most mutations are harmless, either because they are corrected rapidly by the cell, or because they occur in areas of the DNA where they do not influence any cellular functions to a significant extent. On the other hand, some mutations do give rise to uncontrolled growth of cells and that is because they take place at specific sites in DNA where there are oncogenes (which stimulate cell division) or tumour suppressor genes (which inhibit cell division). The consequence of mutation in either of these types of gene is obvious, it leads to uncontrolled cell growth and this is the basis of a neoplasm or tumour.

Benign and malignant tumours

Tumours can be described as being either benign or malignant. Benign tumours, as the name suggests, are less damaging than malignant

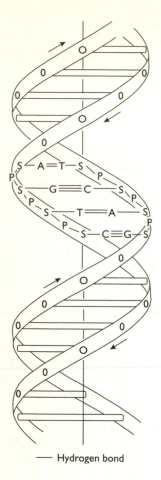

—— Hydrogen bond

Figure 7.1 The quaternary structure of DNA is maintained by hydrogen bonds between the two strands.

tumours. However, they are not entirely harmless as they can grow and exert pressure, for example, in areas of the brain where the resultant pressure may result in the symptoms of stroke or seizures. Nevertheless, in benign tumours the cells are similar to the cells of the tissue in which they have arisen and are described as 'well differentiated'. Benign tumours tend to be slow growing and localised. Malignant tumours, on the other hand, tend to be faster growing, extending beyond the normal margins to invade neighbouring tissue and often contain cells that are not at all like the cells in the tissues where the cancer is located; they are described as 'poorly differentiated' or 'undifferentiated'. The hisotological grading of a tumour relates to how well or poorly differentiated these cells are (Table 7.1). Malignant cells may spread from their tissue of origin and locate in other tissues, a phenomenon called metastasis. For example, malignant cells may travel from the lung – usually via the lymphatic system or the blood – to become lodged in another tissue such as the brain. This process will be discussed in more detail later in this chapter. It is malignant tumours that we usually associate with the term cancer and these tumours are almost always fatal if not treated. Their danger lies, as their name suggests, in that they grow rapidly, overtake the growth of normal cells and spread to areas of the body other than the one in which they have arisen. They invade other tissues and they use the nutritional resources of the body that are destined for healthy cells. In short, malignant tumours are dangerous and debilitating.

Table 7.1 Differences between benign and malignant tumours

	Benign	Malignant
Cells	Relatively normal and mature.	Little resemblance to normal; poorly differentiated, atypical in size and shape, non-uniform and immature.
Growth	Slow and restricted. Non-invasive of surrounding tissue; expansive, pushing aside normal tissue.	Usually rapid and unrestricted. Invasive of surrounding tissue.
Spread	Remains localized. Usually encapsulated.	Metastasizes via blood and lymph streams.
Recurrence	Rarely recurs.	Frequently recurs.
Threat to host	Prognosis favourable. The effect depends on the size and location. May cause pressure on vital organs or obstruct a passageway, which is usually corrected by surgical excision of neoplasm.	Threatens life by reason of its local destructive proliferation and formation of secondary neoplasms in other structures. Prognosis more favourable with early diagnosis and treatment, when cells show less departure from the normal and there is no metastasis.

What causes cancer?

If the causes of cancer were fully understood then, arguably, effective cures would be available. As it is, there are probably several factors conspiring to cause cancer and treatment is mainly aimed, therefore, at removing the cancer or killing the cancer cells by means that will be discussed below. As described above, cancer is essentially a disorder arising in our genetic material. It is likely, therefore, that cancer can be inherited and, indeed, there is some evidence for this. However, caution is required in interpreting such evidence, as the other factors that cause cancer will undoubtedly interact with any genetic predisposition. Environmental factors are undoubtedly linked to cancer and these are the many chemicals in the atmosphere due to pollution and possibly from our efforts at self-pollution through such activities as smoking. The link between cigarette smoking and lung cancer is strong and the link between skin cancer and the prolonged use of certain chemicals is also well established. Radiation, which can be harnessed to good effect in the treatment of cancer, is also known to cause cancer and this includes radiation from the sun, which is a leading cause of skin cancer. Finally, infection by viruses, known as oncogenic viruses, may cause cancer in humans; they have certainly been demonstrated to cause cancer in animals.

Why do these things cause cancer?

All of the above cause cancer because they have the ability to give rise to mutations in the genetic material, DNA. A genetic predisposition to cancer may arise due to inherited factors that make mutations in DNA more likely. These factors could include poor repair mechanisms for damaged DNA or genetic sequences that make the stimulation of onco-genes or the inhibition of tumour suppressor genes more likely. Chemicals may enter the body and interact with DNA directly or may react with other chemicals in the body and with oxygen to give rise to free radicals. Free radicals are highly reactive molecules and atoms and many of these are derived from oxygen. They react with other chemicals in the body, mostly with no adverse effects, but their reaction with DNA can lead to mutations that are carcinogenic (cancer causing). Radiation from radioactive substances can penetrate the protective layer of skin and lead to carcinogenic mutations in DNA. Sunlight contains ultraviolet radiation and this is harmful to the outer layer of the skin where it gives rise to skin cancer but exposure to such things as X-rays can lead to cancer in the deeper tissues of the body. Viruses may lead to cancer because of the way in which they reproduce: viruses are dependent upon the DNA of their host in order to reproduce and the viral DNA becomes incorporated into the host DNA. Some viral DNA may be similar to oncogenes and stimulate the cell to divide in an uncontrolled way. This will be beneficial to the virus as it will rapidly provide more cells containing the virus and, thereby, more copies of the virus. However, it will be harmful to the host infected with the virus.

How can cancer be avoided?

It is not always known what causes specific cancers and it is often not entirely clear what we should be avoiding or, alternatively, doing in order to avoid cancer. However, much attention and effort is expended on this, and we will look at some of the logic behind the health-promoting measures aimed at avoiding cancer. Clearly, if you have a genetic predisposition to developing cancer then there is, at least at this time, absolutely nothing that you can do about that predisposition. However, a disposition to cancer may mean that cancer will not develop unless you impose upon yourself or are exposed to particular environmental triggers. One message for the individual who may be predisposed to cancer is not to smoke cigarettes as the relationship between cigarette smoking and cancer, especially lung cancer, is strong. Nevertheless, it is good advice not to smoke cigarettes whether or not you have a predisposition to cancer. Diet is also implicated in causing and protecting against cancer. Those food items considered 'healthy' tend not to cause cancer and may offer some protection. Those foods considered 'unhealthy' – mostly the enjoyable foods we learn to love as children – are considered to contribute to the risk of cancer. Generally, the 'healthy' group contains vegetables and fruits and the 'unhealthy' group contains sweet foods and foods with a high fat content. Of course, there are reasons other than cancer to consider when changing to a healthy diet such as avoidance of obesity and coronary heart disease.

The reasons why a healthy diet may play a part in causing and preventing cancer is because some foods contain chemicals that are carcinogenic and some foods will develop carcinogenic chemicals when they are cooked – for example, food that is cooked and burned on a barbecue. Such food is shown to contain high levels of cancer-causing chemicals and there is some evidence that diets high in such foods are associated with the development of cancer.

Foods that are considered to protect against cancer contain chemicals that are thought to help to 'mop up' free radicals generated from many metabolic processes in the body and arguably, along with other disorders, linked with the development of cancer. These chemicals include some vitamins found in fresh fruit and vegetables. Fresh fruit and vegetables are considered most effective because cooking destroys many of these vitamins and, again, there is evidence linking diet and protection against cancer – people who eat more fruit and vegetables, with vegetarians at least risk – seem to be at less risk of developing cancer. It is worth noting the language used above which includes the terms 'linking' and 'risk'. It is not possible to establish a direct link between any normal part of our diet and cancer and, likewise, no absolute guarantee that eating a healthy diet will protect against cancer absolutely – it may merely reduce the risk.

On the other hand, the link between exposure to sunshine and skin cancer is very strong. This evidence comes from the fact that people living in sunnier climates have an increased risk of developing skin cancer, and this includes people who move from a temperate to a sunny climate. Also, people with more pigmented skin are at a lower risk of developing skin cancer and this is because the pigment melanin, which is responsible for the phenomenon of sun tan and which is present in higher amounts in the skin of black as opposed to white people, protects against the harmful effects of exposure to sun. There is a greater awareness of the harmful effects of sunshine on skin and more advice is available about covering up areas likely to be affected and using sunlight-blocking creams, especially on young children. Sunbathing, even with the use of sun-blocking creams, is definitely not recommended but is still a widespread activity. People are recommended to bring to the attention of their doctor any changes in their skin that may be due to the effects of sun. Skin cancers may be relatively easily removed but if not removed early enough, they can be as dangerous as any other form of cancer.

Other forms of radiation are also carcinogenic and these come from a variety of sources such as radioactive chemicals and X-ray machinery. Few people are exposed to radioactive chemicals but exposure to X-rays is not uncommon due to their use in diagnosis and screening for disease. Such exposure poses little risk but repeated exposure to X-rays over short periods of time can be potentially harmful and will only be used if the benefit of diagnosing and treating life-threatening conditions outweighs the risk. Staff who work with X-rays – some almost exclusively such as radiographers and radiologists – and nurses who are exposed on occasions, such as accompanying a patient for an X-ray examination, are also at risk. Such workers wear protective clothing – usually lead aprons to protect the body and shield themselves behind leaded areas when operating X-ray machinery. Those who work regularly with radioactivity wear special badges containing detectors that are examined regularly in order to ensure that they are not being over-exposed to X-rays.

Defence against cancer

The body probably has in-built mechanisms to defend against cancer. In fact, given the chemicals to which we are exposed and the fact that oxygen is a very toxic substance, it is surprising that cancer is not more common. It would suggest that such defence mechanisms are both present and effective. Cancerous changes probably quite frequently arise at the genetic and cellular levels and the existence of enzymes in cells that correct mutations in DNA has already been mentioned. However, if genetic mutations do take place and are not detected or corrected by these mechanisms, then cancerous cells will be produced. It is probable that there is a cellular defence mechanism against these abnormal cells involving the immune system. Indeed, it has been suggested that the immune system 'surveys' the body for abnormal cells and then destroys them, a system referred to as immune surveillance. The evidence for this comes from the fact that people who have their immune system suppressed are more prone to the development of cancer. The cells thought to be involved in immune surveillance include the B and T lymphocytes, the natural killer cells and macrophages.

The effects of cancer on the body

Cancer can arise anywhere in the body but does so more commonly in some areas than others. Cancer of the lungs is common in cigarette smokers and breast cancer and prostate cancer are more common in women and men, respectively, than other cancers (Figure 7.2). Nevertheless, cancer does arise in other areas of the body such as the brain and the kidney. Particular tumours are classified (albeit not entirely satisfactorily) according to their site of origin, for example, a muscle tumour is a myosarcoma, a blood vessel tumour is an angioma and a nervous tissue tumour is a neurblastoma. However, within these classifications there are some sub-classifications depending on the precise location of the tumour.

There are many effects of cancer but these can be considered as those that are local to the area where the cancer has arisen and those that arise from metastases elsewhere in the body. As explained above, cancer cells

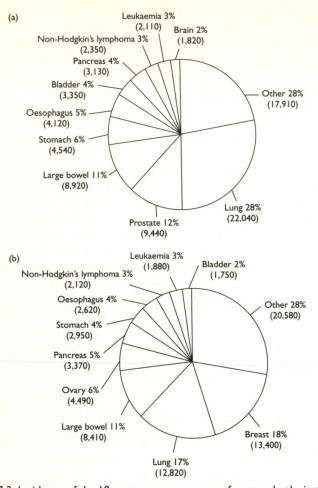

(a)

Leukaemia 3%
(2,110)

Brain 2%
(1,820)

Non-Hodgkin's lymphoma 3%
(2,350)

Pancreas 4%
(3,130)

Bladder 4%
(3,350)

Oesophagus 5%
(4,120)

Stomach 6%
(4,540)

Large bowel 11%
(8,920)

Prostate 12%
(9,440)

Lung 28%
(22,040)

Other 28%
(17,910)

(b)

Leukaemia 3%
(1,880)

Bladder 2%
(1,750)

Non-Hodgkin's lymphoma 3%
(2,120)

Oesophagus 4%
(2,620)

Stomach 4%
(2,950)

Pancreas 5%
(3,370)

Ovary 6%
(4,490)

Large bowel 11%
(8,410)

Lung 17%
(12,820)

Breast 18%
(13,400)

Other 28%
(20,580)

Figure 7.2 Incidence of the 10 most common causes of cancer deaths in the UK in 1997 (Cancer Research Campaign (1999) Cancer Stats: mortality CRC, London). (a) Men; total number of cancers = 79,730. (b) Women; total number of cancers = 74,390. Variations in the cancer mortality between the sexes reflect, as well as anatomical differences, different behavioural and environmental factors. For example, the prevalence of lung cancer in men reflects the fact that many men began to smoke during World War I; the result was a rapid increase in lung cancer in these men, who are now elderly. Women began to smoke in large numbers during World War II; hence, lung cancer in women has begun to overtake breast cancer in incidence. In Scotland this has already occurred.

are unlike the normal cells of a tissue: they have no function within the tissue where they originate but they grow more rapidly than the normal cells and quickly invade the tissue. Cancer cells lose the contact inhibition displayed by normal cells that stops normal cells growing when they come into contact with other cells and cancer cells may also secrete enzymes that digest surrounding normal tissue and help them to invade it. Depending upon where the cancer has arisen a tumour may invade other nearby tissues but the usual way in which it spreads is by metastasis via the lymphatic system, the blood stream, the serous cavities or in the cerebrospinal fluid.

Metastases

The lymphatic tissue, which is made up of capillaries, nodes and large vessels, is ubiquitous in the body, except in the head. As previously described, the purpose of the lymphatic system is to return excess tissue fluid to the bloodstream. However, the lymphatic tissue is also very effective at taking cancer cells that break off tumours in one tissue to other tissues (Figure 7.3). One particular cancer that spreads via the lymphatic vessels is breast cancer. Breast tissue is modified lymphatic tissue and, therefore, is linked closely to the lymphatic tissue. In fact, it is possible to 'stage' the spread of breast cancer by investigating the extent to which the nodes in the lymphatic system have been involved.

Some cancer cells are deposited in the bloodstream by the lymphatic system and other cancer cells get into the bloodstream by breaking off tumours that have eroded blood vessels. In the cavities of the body the presence of cancer increases the production of serous fluid and this removes cells from tumours and deposits them elsewhere in the serous cavities. Finally, tumours arising in the central nervous system may spread elsewhere through the cerebrospinal fluid that bathes the brain and spinal cord. For instance, tumours in the brain may spread to the spinal cord. As with the spread to the lymphatic nodes the presence of metastases establishes the particular 'stage' of the disease.

In fact, metastases most commonly spread to the lungs, the bones, the brain and the liver and this may have occurred before a diagnosis of cancer has been made. Clearly, the extent to which metastases have spread is inversely related to the survival of the person with cancer and early diagnosis of cancer, if at all possible, is desirable.

Tumours have a wide range of detrimental effects wherever they occur and these range from direct physical effects to those that are involved with homeostatic imbalance. For example, as tumours grow they will

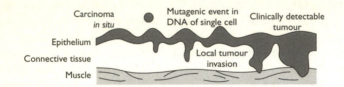

Carcinoma *in situ*

Mutagenic event in DNA of single cell

Clinically detectable tumour

Epithelium

Connective tissue

Muscle

Local tumour invasion

Lymphatic spread

Tumour cells penetrate local lymphatic vessels

Cells then spread to nearby lymph nodes

Thoracic lymph duct empties tumour cells into blood

Anteriovenous spread

Tumour cells enter and travel in blood

The cells become enmeshed in nearest capillary network

The tumour cells reach, for example, liver sinusoid and grow in liver substance

Liver metastases become established

Serous spread

For example, in lung tumour, cells penetrate pleura, cause irritation and excess pleural fluid

Widespresad metastatic deposits spread by seeding. Excess fluid forms malignant pleural effusion and lung may collapse

CSF spread

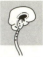

Tumour cells may travel in the cerebrospinal fluid along the spinal cord to the brain

Figure 7.3 The cancer process.

exert pressure on tissues around them such as nerves, blood vessels and hollow organs with obvious effects. A tumour exerting pressure on a nerve will cause loss of sensation and possibly function in the affected part of the body; a tumour exerting pressure on a blood vessel will lead to ischaemia of the area supplied by the blood vessel and a tumour exerting pressure on the oesophagus will cause difficulty with swallowing (dysphagia). Some tumours will outgrow the normal tissue and, thereby, prevent the tissue from carrying out its normal function, for example, secretion and absorption in the gastrointestinal tract. Other tumours may invade the blood vessels surrounding them leading to bleeding and this can be life-threatening in itself if major blood vessels are involved. Tumours require a high blood supply, which deprives surrounding tissue of blood supply leading to necrosis (death) of normal tissue. The tumour may infiltrate the skin (fungate) and will be susceptible to infection. Tumours in bone marrow will reduce the production of blood cells that help to fight infection and this, coupled with other aspects of cancer such as poor nutrition, will also lead to a susceptibility to infection. Certain tumours, for example, of the pancreas, liver and kidneys will lead to metabolic imbalances leading to lack of homeostasis in such things as glucose metabolism and fluid and electrolyte balance. Invasion of bone tissue by tumours, either a primary site or as a result of metastases, will lead to breakdown of bone tissue and release of calcium into the blood and hypercalcaemia leading to serious effects of nausea, vomiting and potential renal failure.

There are other effects of cancer on the body at sites removed from the tumour and include blood cell abnormalities, nerve and muscle cell degeneration including the brain, pyrexia and disturbances to the endocrine system and metabolism. Many cancer patients suffer cachexia, which literally means a 'bad state' and is manifested in muscle wastage, emaciation and generalised weakness. This effect appears to be due to metabolic disturbance such that the basal metabolic rate is increased while digestion and absorption of nutrients is decreased. Cancer is clearly a considerable threat to homeostasis.

Treating cancer

Surgery is one option for some forms of cancer where the tumour is localised, accessible and where removal is not liable to cause a poorer immediate outcome for the surrounding tissues that might threaten survival. Clearly, not all tumours are amenable to surgery and where metastases have occurred, surgery may prolong a patient's life by removing a primary, life-threatening tumour but cannot deal with all the possible sites in the body to which the cancer may have spread. Where surgery is not an option, and often as an adjunct to surgery, then there are two other main strategies for treating cancer and these involve radiotherapy and chemotherapy, sometimes used together.

Radiotherapy involves focusing beams of X-rays at tumours in an attempt to kill the cancer cells and leave most of the surrounding tissue intact. We have already seen that X-rays can be dangerous but also how they are used for diagnostic purposes. In radiotherapy for cancer several relatively non-harmful doses of X-ray irradiation are aimed at a tumour from different angles and where they converge the dose is high enough to kill the cancer cells. Other tissues through which the X-rays travel are left relatively unaffected. However, exposure to X-rays for the treatment of cancer is for considerably longer periods than for diagnostic purposes and the levels are monitored very closely and only administered to the patient over several short sessions. Radiotherapy is also used following surgery in a more generalised way to prevent the spread of cancer. For example, following the removal of a breast tumour the area may be irradiated with the intention of killing any remaining cancer cells, which, growing more rapidly, are more susceptible to the radiation than the healthy tissue.

Chemotherapy also makes use of the differences between tumours and normal cells and attempts, respectively, to kill cancer cells and to leave healthy cells unaffected. Chemotherapy is not aimed at cancer cells in the same way as radiotherapy; the drugs are usually administered intravenously thereby exposing the whole body to their effects. There are various chemotherapeutic agents and while they all aim to kill the more rapidly growing cancer cells they all have an effect on normal cells and especially on those that grow rapidly such as the cells that line the mouth, the cells that line the gastrointestinal tract and the hair follicles. It is the effects on these tissues during chemotherapy that cause the common side-effects of nausea and vomiting and hair loss.

Conclusion

Cancer is a disease of genetic origin. Mutations arise in DNA spontaneously or as a result of chemical or radiation damage. Some cancer may be caused by viruses. The essential feature of cancer is that it leads to uninhibited cell division, giving rise either to tumours or spread of abnormal cells throughout the body. Some forms of cancer can be very localised and, thereby, relatively easily treated. Other forms of cancer, malignant forms, tend to spread from their site of origin to other areas of the body. Some people are more disposed towards cancer than others and this may be a result of both genetic and environmental factors. The treatment of cancer, other than by surgery, depends on killing cancer cells – using radiation or chemicals – more quickly than the normal cells of the body. Treating cancer in this way can give rise to problems in other tissues that also divide rapidly such as the lining of the gastrointestinal tract and the hair follicles. Essentially, cancer arises from a disorder in homeostasis of cell division and has profound homeostatic consequences for the whole of the body.

Questions

1   What are the common features of all cancers?
2   Explain how cancer can be seen as a disease of genetic origin?
3   Compare and contrast benign and malignant tumours.
4   How does the body defend itself against cancer?
5   If you are genetically predisposed to developing cancer does that mean that you will develop it? What factors should be taken into account?
6   How can the unique features of cancer determine modes of treatment? Can you explain the side-effects of chemotherapy?

Chapter 8

Stress, shock and pain

Aim

To understand how stress, shock and pain are deviations from homeostasis.

Learning outcomes

This chapter should enable the reader to:

- understand the physiology of stress;
- describe and explain the causes and manifestations of shock;
- demonstrate an insight into the phenomenon of pain, its assessment and alleviation.

Introduction

This chapter brings together three concepts, which, while they may all occur simultaneously, are not necessarily directly related to one another. Stress, shock and pain all represent outcomes of deviations from normal – from homeostasis – in the body. Stress is the physiological result of either a physiological or psychological stressor (things that cause stress). Shock is the pathophysiological outcome of an extreme disturbance to the cardiovascular system, again the result of either a physiological or psychological stressor. Pain is a complex psychological and physiological process that is in itself is both a stressor and the response to a stressor. Each of these phenomena will be considered in turn; the causes, the consequences and the possible approaches to their alleviation. In stress, shock and pain the nurse has important roles to play and these will be highlighted alongside each.

Stress

Stress is considered as the body's reaction to environmental changes and challenges and, therefore, is part of normal functioning and integral to life. In moderate degrees, stress arouses and alerts us, improving and enhancing mental and physical activity. Therefore, despite the popular connotation, stress is not necessarily a bad thing. When we suffer from stress it is when the demands put on the body, from whatever source, exceed the resources to cope disrupting our general equilibrium and causing distress.

Only exceptional people will never have experienced what is commonly referred to as 'stress' these days. An expression that one is 'stressed' is usually taken to indicate a negative reaction to events and circumstances but stress has a wider meaning in sociological, psychological and biological terms. Sociologically, stress refers to the circumstances in which individuals find themselves which might produce stress such as work pressure, changing jobs or houses and experiencing crises such as bereavement. Psychologically, sources of stress refer to emotional states often the result of interpersonal problems, frustrations or a perceived sense of being powerless. Biologically, stress can mean any deviation from normal, that is, from homeostasis and this can arise from actual stressful situations, as might be described sociologically, but also from perceived stressful situations as might arise psychologically – even in the absence of stressful circumstances. Biologically, stress may mean physical injury, dehydration or extremes of temperature but there are also, probably, biological outcomes from sociological and psychological stress that will also be considered below. While it is important to understand the above distinctions, for the purposes of this chapter, stress will be considered as a concept with both psychosocial and biological causes and consequences.

Clearly, in order to avoid stress we take many actions such as avoiding injury, eating, drinking and keeping warm, ensuring adequate income and maintaining harmonious communication. In some situations, however, there is little that we can do about the stress that arises such as extreme events in life that we all are likely to experience. However, it is worth noting that the stress that we so readily refer to these days and that seems to be present in many lives may also be a motivating factor. Research has demonstrated, for instance, in occupations where stress is high such as the job of consultant surgeon, the same things which could cause stress are the very things which bring most satisfaction to the surgeons such as working under pressure and achieving long lists of operations. There are many who confess to needing a constant 'adrenaline rush' in both their working and recreational lives. However, for most of us, in order to avoid stress, we try to organise our lives. For example, we may get to work early in order to get through the work demands of the day, stay longer in order to do the same or, more effectively, we learn not to 'bite off more than we can chew'.

What is stress?

Whenever a concept is poorly understood then theories and models will abound about its true nature and stress provides a perfect example. Models of stress consider stress from four perspectives: the stimulus-based, the response-based, the transactional and the phenomenological. Such theories and models have not been considered up to his point in the book but if readers are going to explore stress further then they will need to know the significance of the different models and which are applicable to nursing practice. The stimulus-based model of stress considers that people are exposed continually to stressors and these can range from the mundane such as having a heavy workload or the common cold, to the more serious end of the spectrum such as serious illness or getting divorced. While the model accurately describes generally agreed sources of stress, it fails to explain how some people cope with stress better than others – as they clearly do. The approach to reducing stress under this model is to remove stressful stimuli and, while this is possible to some extent and some circumstances, it is clearly impossible in others – such as being or becoming disabled, severely ill or bereaved. The response-based model of stress is really the other side of the coin from the stimulus-based model in that stress is seen in terms of the experience of a person, their actual response to perceived threat. This is reasonable as we can never really know if someone is stressed unless there is a detectable stress response. The way in which the person perceives the stressor (the cognitive-affective domain) triggers neurological and physiological reactions to the stressor. How the individual person copes with the stress will vary but will be by means of manipulating the environment to reduce the source of the stress response or by means of making some cognitive or affective adjustments. If that is unsuccessful the person may suffer from detrimental effects on target organs whereby the normal homeostatic function can be impaired by the physiological effects of the stress response. This model is helpful because it incorporates the physical reactions to stress and offers an explanation for why stress may be detrimental. It also incorporates the concept of coping with stress.

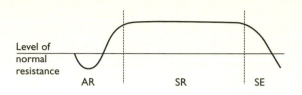

Figure 8.1 The general adaptation syndrome. AR, alarm reaction; SR, stage of resistance; SE, stage of exhaustion.

However, one of the best known theories of stress is the general adaptation syndrome (GAS) of Hans Seyle (Figure 8.1). Selye contends that, regardless of the nature of the stressor, the body will respond physiologically in three distinct stages, the alarm reaction of 'fight fright and flight', the stage of resistance and if the stressor is overwhelming, the stage of exhaustion. This has considerable currency for physiological stressors such as injury or extremes of heat and cold but does not explain so well the psychological responses to stress. The transactional model of stress is perhaps the model with most currency, not only due to its ability to explain the phenomenon of stress but because its usefulness for those who help people in stressful situations such as psychologists, nurses and counsellors. This model, proposed by Lazarus and Folkman, envisages individuals in a continual process of appraising their situation in terms of its stressfulness. Only if the situation is perceived as stressful would a stress response be triggered. This is seen as primary appraisal. Secondary appraisal is then made to determine the coping strategy to be adopted. Thus, within this model it is recognised that individuals appraise situations differently respond to them differently and adopt different coping strategies, some better than others! This model has proved helpful in the management of stress because it realises that each person is different and that they can be helped not only in terms of the appraisal of potentially stressful situations but also in terms of securing the most appropriate coping strategy.

Finally, there is a phenomenological approach to stress that looks at stress within the context in which people find themselves and rests largely on the experiences of stress described as meaningful by the individual. This is not that far removed from the transactional model of stress and also helps to explain why some people view certain circumstances as stressful while others seem unaffected. Of course, there are people who do not seem to suffer from stress a great deal or who seem to cope extremely well with stressful events and stressful situations and these people are described as being resilient. However, stress management and associated interventions by nurses and others is usually for individuals who tend not to have this resilience and who may benefit from learning some of the techniques that naturally resilient people may apply to potentially stressful events and situations.

What does stress feel like?

I am sure that each reader could offer some answers to this but the real point of this section is to look for common experiences of stress and to explain why we feel like we do when we are 'stressed'.

Essentially, stress is a state of arousal and preparedness for adverse circumstances, described by Seyle in the alarm 'fight fright and flight' reaction (Table 8.1). This state arises from an increase in the activity of the sympathetic nervous system, part of the autonomic or involuntary nervous system, and the effects on the body include increased heart rate, deep breathing, sweating, a dry mouth and decreased motility in the digestive tract ('tightening of the stomach' in lay terms) all of which may be felt by the person under stress. There are also other effects that are less tangible such as an increase in blood glucose levels. All of these effects arise from the effect of stress on the sympathetic nervous system and the adrenal medulla, which produce adrenaline and noradrenaline, and subsequently on the endocrine adrenal cortex, which secretes corticosteroids. The purpose of the alarm 'fight or flight' response is to mobilise physiological resources to deal with the perceived threat to the body's integrity and these acute, or short-term effects of stress and the fight or flight reaction are clearly useful if, in fact, you have to fight or flee a dangerous situation. Once the situation has been fled or altered then the fight or flight reaction will subside. However, in the twenty-first century, the stressors experienced often do not require physical fighting or flight and the mobilised resources are not utilised. This is of particular concern in prolonged chronic as opposed to acute stress, when the equally prolonged nervous and, more particularly, the endocrine reaction continues and becomes maladaptive and will eventually lead to the adverse effects of stress on the body and mind. The detrimental effects result, for the most part, from excessive and prolonged levels of corticosteroids from the adrenal cortex and these include muscle wastage, thinning of the skin, reduced immune response and delayed wound healing. In this way it can be seen that uncontained stress will eventually disturb homeostasis. If the stressor is totally unrelenting, the nervous and endocrine systems will eventually cease to respond adequately to any stress and the ability of the person to cope with stress diminishes and this can be manifest through such things as physical debility, specific disorder or disease, anxiety, depression and burnout. Clearly, stress can be harmful.

The harmful effects of stress

Optimal adaptive stress that helps us cope with what life's ongoing challenges has been described as 'eustress'. However, as indicated, prolonged stress – either because the source of the stress is not removed or the person is unable to cope with the stress – leads to exhaustion and in this state we are not able to function effectively. Stress is commonly associated with migraine, anxiety and depression and although none of these is solely caused by stress, stress may precipitate them all in vulnerable individuals. It is hard to define precisely the relationship between stress and depression as people who are depressed may also, subsequently, suffer from stress. Anxiety, the emotion almost used synonymously with stress, may be exhibited as panic attacks with symptoms of extreme sympathetic nervous system stimulation – palpitations, sweating and hyperventilation. Stress is also associated with syndromes of post-traumatic stress disorder and chronic fatigue syndrome. Both of these disorders are poorly understood and some experts even dispute their existence. Nevertheless, stressful situations can lead to the flashbacks that are characteristic of post-traumatic stress disorder and as the outcome of chronic stress can be exhaustion, there is good reason to believe that chronic fatigue and stress may be linked.

Stress and disease

The list of diseases with which stress is associated is long and ranges from cardiovascular disease to cancer and includes such things as autoimmune diseases and infections. The link to cardiovascular disease may be through the extreme and prolonged sympathetic stimulation that occurs with stress (Table 8.2). This is likely to have an adverse effect on the heart and the blood vessels leading to such things as angina and hypertension and on the integrity of the gastric mucosa. Prolonged stress leading to raised corticosteroid levels may account for precipitating atheromatous deposits in blood vessels and be equally detrimental to the gastric mucosa. Prolonged elevation of corticosteroids also results in a suppression of the immune system leading to infections and arguably autoimmune disorders such as rheumatoid arthritis and diabetes mellitus

Table 8.1 Physical signs (including common clinical measurements) and symptoms which any occur in acute stress

Site	Physiological basis	Physical signs and common clinical measurements	Physical symptoms
Cardiovascular system	Increased cardiac rate and output	Tachycardia Pulse of full volume Raised blood pressure	Pounding heart Palpitations Chest pain Headache
Respiratory system	CNS arousal If the hyperventilation is not in response to physiological need, low pp CO_2 results and leads to vasodilatation, fall in blood pressure and, in extreme cases, tetany	Increased rate and depth of ventilation Tetany in extreme cases	Dizziness, faintness, panic (in extreme cases) Tingling in the extremities Muscle spasm (in extreme cases)
Gastrointestinal system	Reduced blood supply to and reduced secretion in gastrointestinal tract Decreased or increased mobility of tract	Vomiting Diarrhoea Constipation Anorexia or overeating	Dry mouth Indigestion/dyspepsia Nausea Diarrhoea (often frequent) Constipation Anorexia or overeating

Skin	Contraction of pilomotor muscles	Erection of hair	Clammy palms
	Cholinergic sweating	Sweating	
	Reduced blood supply	Pallor	
Eye	Contraction of radial muscle	Dilated pupils	Blurred vision
Muscle	CNS arousal	Muscle tension, tremor	Headache
		Muscle spasm in severe cases	Muscle tension, tremor, twitching
		Lack of coordination	Lack of coordination
			Back pain
General	CNS arousal	Insomnia	Insomnia
		Restlessness	Restlessness
	Increased metabolic rate	Low-grade pyrexia	Fatigue/weakness
			Feeling hot or cold

Source: Boore, JRP, Champion R & Ferguson M (1987) *Nursing the Physically ill Adult*. Churchill Livingstone, Edinburgh.

Table 8.2 Some diseases in which stress is or may be an aetiological factor

Coronary heart disease	Cerebrovascular accident
Hypertension	Migraine
Bronchial asthma	Peptic ulceration
Ulcerative colitis	Spastic colon
Diabetes mellitus	Hyperthyroidism
Reproductive disorders	Growth retardation
Rheumatoid arthritis	Multiple sclerosis
Eczema and dermatitis	Cancer
Autoimmune disease	Allergies
Infections	

and even cancer. In none of the above is there a direct link between the diseases and stress and it is possible that other factors lead to both stress and these diseases in vulnerable individuals. It has also been suggested that in unrelenting conditions of stress when the homeostatic mechanisms move from being excessive to a more central failure at pituitary level, there may be some fertility problems and 'failure to thrive' in children suffering severe emotional or physical deprivation.

Managing stress

Some people just seem to manage stress on their own and even if they suffer from it, as many claim, they do not appear to require help. On the other hand, some people simply cannot cope with what may be generally thought of a low levels of stress and may quickly run out of resources and seek help, often from the family doctor or, if available, occupational health departments. Coping mechanisms can be divided into two categories: direct action and indirect palliative action. In direct action, active steps are taken to demolish, avoid or flee from the threatening situation. Equally, direct action may involve constructive, problem-solving strategies. Indirect methods tend to be concerned with reducing the unpleasant emotions experienced, even though the actual source of stress may not (at that particular time) be addressed. Emotion-focused strategies may take the form of sedative medication, alcohol, relaxation techniques or the use of defence mechanisms.

The range of options for helping people cope with stress are varied and may simply involve a period of rest or, following a period of rest, returning the person to a less stressful situation. Some people find therapy helpful and a range of options from counselling to behavioural therapy is available. In extreme cases people may require more specific medication and this may be just something to help them to sleep in order to overcome the exhausting effects of stress, avoid anxiety and panic attacks, and cope with their work or deal with developing symptoms of depression.

Shock

The term 'shock', like stress, is used frequently but, unlike stress – which is relatively common – it is unlikely, despite the colloquial use of the term, that many people have really experienced shock. Shock, which, of course, is an extreme stressor on the body, is a life-threatening condition and its essential feature is a lack of perfusion of tissues with blood leading to lack of oxygen supply to the tissues and a failure to remove waste products. Shock is a common cause of death and arises for many reasons. However, the most common cause of shock is due to massive loss of blood or plasma (hypovolaemic shock) and this may follow severe trauma such as from a road traffic accident or a gunshot wound. Shock also occurs when the heart does not function properly as in a myocardial infarction (cardiogenic shock) and for other reasons, collectively known as distributive shock, whereby there is collapse of the vasculature, for example, in septic shock, neurogenic shock and anaphylactic shock. These will be considered in more detail below.

Shock is an excellent example of a condition where the homeostatic mechanisms of the body may restore equilibrium or work to their limits and yet be overwhelmed and fail to cope. This can be seen in the stages of shock. The first, or initial, stage of shock is not detectable from signs and symptoms but due to the disturbance to homeostasis and the lack of tissue perfusion the cells begin to metabolise without oxygen leading to the production of lactic acid and an increase in the acid levels in the blood (Figure 8.2).

The next stage is the compensatory stage in which the homeostatic mechanisms of the body that respond to lack of tissue perfusion by detecting a fall in blood pressure, the fall in oxygen levels and the concomitant fall in blood pH and try to compensate. This compensation has nervous, hormonal and chemical components: the nervous system reacts in a 'fight or flight' manner via the sympathetic nervous system and initiates a widespread (but selective) vasoconstrictive response in order to maintain the blood supply to the vital organs while restricting it from, at this time, non-vital tissue such as the skin, digestive tract and even

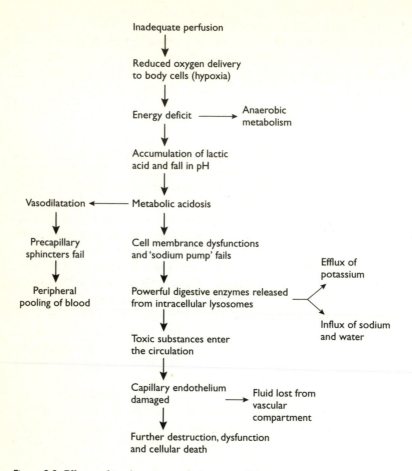

Figure 8.2 Effects of inadequate perfusion on cell function.

initially the kidneys. The person in shock will look pale and feel cold and clammy as a result. In addition, the neuroendocrine system is stimulated to release adrenaline, noradrenaline and corticosteroids – the stress response discussed in an earlier section. The lowered level of oxygen in the blood is detected by the chemoreceptors and this chemical signal stimulates the respiratory system. The person in shock will hyperventilate and blow off carbon dioxide as a means of restoring to normal the blood pH, but also resulting in respiratory alkalosis. The stress response associated with the experience of shock will exacerbate the above reactions.

If the cause of the shock is not corrected and overwhelms the ability of the compensatory mechanisms, the body moves into what is known as the progressive stage of shock with potential widespread deleterious effects on the body. If this stage is not corrected a vicious cycle is established whereby the initial vasoconstrictive consequences of the shock, if not successful in restoring homeostasis, result in collapse of the vasculature that initiates yet further (desperate) 'corrective' vasoconstriction and yet more severe signs and symptoms. Essentially, the tissues of the body will become depleted of oxygen and will be unable to carry out their normal functions and this may lead, amongst other things, to kidney failure, cerebral anoxia and cardiac arrest. In the later stages of shock when cellular derangement has set in, toxins are released into the blood that damage the vessels of the microcirculation such that fluid is lost from the vascular compartment. The low levels of fluid in the cardiovascular system will lead to aggregation of erythrocytes to form microclots that paradoxically use up the body's clotting factors in a vain attempt to restore equilibrium and bleeding can occur, a condition known as disseminated intravascular coagulation. In the digestive tract, ischaemic destruction may result in bacteria entering the blood and similar damage in the lungs damages the delicate alveolar-capillary network causing respiratory distress, 'shock' lung. The diminished cerebral perfusion will lead to slower responses and increasingly reduced level of consciousness. Finally, if shock is not dealt with in the progressive stage the refractory (resistant to intervention) stage will ensue when it becomes impossible to reverse the signs and symptoms of shock, and this will lead to mortal cardiac failure and death.

The causes of shock

The types of shock have been outlined above and they all have different causes. Hypovolaemic shock, literally shock caused by a low volume of fluid in the cardiovascular system, may be caused by bleeding either externally, which will usually be easy to recognise, but also by internal bleeding where there will not be the obvious signs that bleeding is taking place. Other causes of hypovolaemic shock include major burns and severe diarrhoea and vomiting. This may occur after trauma or when a blood vessel in a compromised gastrointestinal tract ruptures and bleeding will occur into the internal cavities of the body. Prolonged diarrhoea or vomiting, where there is a large loss of fluid from the gastrointestinal tract, or burns to large areas of the body, where there is a large loss of plasma fluid from the surface of the burn, will also lead to shock.

In cardiogenic shock, which may follow a myocardial infarction, the heart fails as a pump, the cardiac output drops and shock ensues. Distributive shock occurs for four different reasons. Septic shock follows infection by certain pathogens, which, as well as directly damaging the myocardium and therefore cardiac output, release toxins into the blood, which, in an attempt to contain the septicaemia, leads to metabolic and immune system changes that in extremis leads to derangement of the vascular tone, loss of fluid from the vasculature. Commonly in neurogenic shock, trauma to the central nervous system leads to an increase in parasympathetic nervous system activity and widespread vasodilatation, low blood pressure and shock and spinal shock, which arises from damage to the spine, leads to a cessation in the pathways that maintain cardiovascular tone, leading to shock. Fainting (syncope) is also a mild form of neurogenic shock where, for example, the experience of significant emotion can affect the vasomotor centre in the brain leading to loss of vasomotor tone and a temporary episode of cerebral hypoxia. Standing for prolonged periods allowing for pooling of blood in the legs may have similar effect. Homeostatic mechanisms normally correct this effectively. Finally, anaphylactic shock results from an extreme allergic reaction and widespread release of histamine in the body leading to generalised vasodilatation, loss of vascular integrity and shock. In the above serious examples of distributive shock it can be argued that in the end all shock is a form of hypovolaemic shock.

Recognising shock

The cardinal signs of shock are low blood pressure and a rapid pulse. The compensatory mechanisms will result in the shocked person looking pale and feeling cold and clammy with rapid shallow breathing and restless and confused. Due to reduced perfusion of the kidneys, urine output will fall.

Nurses need to be aware of the signs and symptoms of shock in the clinical setting, where monitoring of blood pressure and pulse is routine after procedures, such as surgery, where hypovolaemic shock is a major potential complication. The nurse may be required to recognise shock occurring outside of the clinical areas, for example, in people who collapse following trauma or experience a myocardial infarction in the street, and institute first aid measures. The precise measures will depend upon the cause of the shock but the ABC (airway, breathing and circulation) principles of first aid and basic life support may be sufficient to save or preserve life until help can be summoned and advanced life support measures instituted as necessary. If someone is obviously bleeding then the bleeding should be stemmed by the application of pressure, as explained in Chapter 6. Help should be summoned, using the emergency services, as soon as possible. Meanwhile, the person should be kept calm, warm (but not overheated) and the nurse should monitor overall appearance, pulse and respiratory rate and level of consciousness, trying if possible to maintain consciousness by talking to them.

Pain

Pain is a complex physiological, psychological and sociological phenomenon and one that is impossible to do justice to in a short space. However, the nurse needs to understand the underlying mechanisms of pain and the ways in which pain can be alleviated. It is possible, only to a limited extent, to answer the question of why we experience pain. There are times when pain is useful and protective: when we stub our toe we learn to be careful about where we put our feet; if we bang our heads we learn to duck when there are low objects and if we burn our hand we learn not to pick up hot objects. It only works to some extent as we sometimes do these things again! Pain is also associated with more severe injury, where the experience of pain may prevent aggravating the injury by preventing further movement and again, it may help us to avoid such injury in the future. On the other hand, there are situations where the experience of pain can extend well beyond the point where it has any value. Pain is also associated with certain diseases and a prime example can be seen in certain established cancers where the pain is long lasting and often diffuse, unlike the acute nature of the pain of an injury. Although the physiology of this pain can usually be understood, the purpose behind such pain – which, as suggested, often only occurs long after cancer has been identified – is a mystery. If the pain occurred early it could be taken as a warning signal, but this is not the case and such pain causes prolonged misery, if not alleviated, for cancer sufferers.

Types of pain

Pain is sometime described as being either acute or chronic. A good example of acute pain would be burning a finger on a hot pan, or accidentally cutting yourself with a knife. The pain that is associated with cancer is a prime example of chronic pain. However, the distinction between these two types of pain is not always so distinct: some injuries in which acute pain is experienced can lead to long-term conditions where chronic neuropathic pain is experienced. Back pain resulting from a herniated intervertebral disc in the spine (a 'slipped disc') is a good example of a condition where the initial pain is acute in the extreme but where a lower grade pain may persist for many months proving difficult to relieve effectively.

Pain mechanisms

Pain is a response, by the body, to different types of injury such as mechanical injury, extremes of temperature or chemical injury. Pain is recognised by specific receptors called nociceptors, free sensory nerve endings that form a widespread and overlapping network in almost every tissue of the body. However, they are not ubiquitous. Some parts of the body contain no nociceptors, for example, the lungs and the brain. When tissue is damaged the nerve endings are stimulated by the release of chemicals such as prostaglandins and histamine and once activated an electrical impulse is conducted along afferent neurones to the dorsal horn of the spinal cord where ascending pathways carry the impulses to centres within the brain. This may sound simple but in reality we are increasingly recognisng the complexity and plasticity of the neural pathways involved in pain transmission that may go some way to understanding the challenge on chronic neuropathic pain. The one key theory that has significantly influenced our understanding of pain in the past 35–40 years is the 'gate control' theory of pain, proposed by Melzack and Wall. The original theory was quite simple in concept in that they argued that the transmission of painful stimuli could be controlled by a gating mechanism that they located in the substantia gelatinosa of the dorsal horn. They suggested that when significant number of impulses along the large A-beta fibres carrying signals for touch and warmth, then the transmission of pain impulses carried in the small A-delta and C-fibres is blocked by a synaptic gate. Only when the pain impulses predominated would the gate open and the individual experience pain. However, the modulation of pain does not occur only at the level of the spinal cord. With increasing refinement, the gate control model now incorporates the role of pain inhibiting descending impulses from the cerebral cortex and thalamus. It is thought that these inhibitory impulses, mediated by increasingly better understood neurotransmitters, may be directly under cognitive and emotional control in 'deciding' how much pain an individual will feel.

We will return to the gate control theory below when we look at the alleviation of pain but it is worth pointing out here that the gate control theory is very useful in explaining how certain forms of analgesia (pain relief) works and, indeed, that many of the anatomical features proposed in the gate control theory have been established.

Assessing pain

With very few exceptions, everyone experiences pain at some point in their life. However, describing pain in terms of its location, type and severity is not easy. Nevertheless, nurses have to assess pain in patients in order to know whether it is necessary to administer pain relief, if the condition of the patient is deteriorating or improving and whether or not it is reasonable to ask a patient to move following an operation of traumatic injury. Pain can usually be accurately localised if it is peripheral and somatic (the A-delta fibre transmission), but central visceral pain (C-fibre transmission) is less easily localised and may be very diffuse and ongoing. Pain may also be referred pain from one part of the body to another, a phenomenon that can bemuse the individual. Commonly, the origin of the pain is visceral but the experience is somatic, for example, liver and gall bladder disorder may present with right shoulder tip pain (which can be excruciating) or pain from a cardiac origin may present in the throat or down the left arm. The explanation for this is that the location of the referred pain developed from the same embryonic structure as its visceral origin. A particularly distressing experience is that of phantom pain from an amputated body part, usually a limb. Many explanations, discussed later in this chapter, are put forward to try to explain the experience of pain from a source that is no more. Whatever the type of pain patients will also have some idea of its intensity and may describe their pain as 'burning' or 'crushing' and, certainly, they will know if it is getting better or worse. A number of scales exist to help patients to communicate the location, intensity, pattern and effect of their pain. The intensity, for example, can be rated on numerical rating scale from 1 to 10, by a verbal rating scale or simply on a visual analogue scale where the patient is asked to indicate the point on the scale from 'no pain' to 'worst possible pain' that best reflects what they feel. The nurse should be aware that the experience of pain is very individual and that any ratings made using such scale are merely adjuncts to helping the patient describe their pain and the nurse make the appropriate intervention. Some people have lower thresholds for pain and in some cultures it is more acceptable than others to display the fact that pain is being experienced. Nurses should take pain expressed seriously but should remember that pain is difficult to articulate and many patients, for complex reasons, may not disclose their pain. Pain assessment demands more clinical discernment than might initially be thought. It is well understood that the existence of unrelieved pain may delay recovery. Following surgery, for example, it is usually advisable, for patients' physiological well-being, to start moving as soon as possible. The fact that the presence of pain will inhibit this process reinforces the importance of accurate pain assessment and concomitant optimal means of pain relief as a core to good nursing care. Patients who do not regain movement soon after an operation may not be able to breathe deeply or move the large muscles in their legs and this may lead to complications such as chest infection, pressure area problems and deep vein thrombosis, referred to in Chapter 6.

Alleviating pain

It is possible, in most circumstances, to alleviate pain. A great deal of pain relief is achieved using drugs that are called analgesics. Pain can be dealt with according to the type of pain being experienced. For example, peripheral pain, simple toothache, a sore throat or a burn to a finger can be alleviated using drugs that act at the site of pain and these drugs include aspirin and paracetamol although there are many other drugs used to treat such pain including non-steroidal anti-inflammatory drugs such as ibuprofen. Precisely how these drugs work is very much the subject of current research but they may act generally to reduce the levels of substances such as prostaglandins (by inhibiting the cycloxygense enzymes) released when tissues are injured and which make nociceptors more sensitive to pain mediating substances such as histamine. You will recall from Chapter 3 that paracetamol and aspirin are also used for their antipyretic properties suggesting some common mode of action. Analgesics such as paracetamol and other non-opioid analgesics are not very effective (at least on their own) at alleviating central pain, or pain that is considered moderate or severe, and this is where a class of drugs known as the opiates or opioids work well. Opioid analgesics include drugs such as morphine, fentanyl, codeine and diamorphine (heroin). These drugs act at receptors in the brain and their mode of action is, in part, explained by the gate control theory. By acting at the opioid receptors, particularly μ-receptors, within and outside the central nervous system they may stimulate the descending pathways envisaged by the gate control theory thereby closing the gates to the ascending pain pathways. The gate control theory may also explain why a wide range of methods, not involving drugs, may be effective at relieving pain: essentially, they are working by closing the gates to the pain pathway in the spinal cord. This could explain why many patients find that massage, heat application, TENS (transcutaneous electrical nerve stimulation) and even just being diverted from thinking about pain, work for them. It should be emphasised that patient responses to pain relief tend to be as individualised as their experience of pain.

It is also established that, for the brain to have opioid receptors, the brain must produce its own 'natural opiates' (which are actually small protein or peptide molecules). These are the endorphins and enkephalins, which under certain circumstances act to reduce the sensation of pain and even to elevate mood. The circumstances include exercise, which may explain the 'runners' high' that some athletes feel after prolonged exercise, and may explain why soldiers wounded in battle often feel no pain initially in the heat of the battle.

The use of opioids as analgesics continues to raise anxiety among patients and professionals about addiction. After all, many opioid drugs are used illegally for 'recreational' purposes with devastating effects: they lead to long-term addiction with a range of adverse psychological and physiological effects and can lead to death. However, professionals should be aware, and convey this to patients, that if opioid analgesics are used appropriately then the risk of addiction is very small. In fact, it is considered that when opioids are used as analgesics, while they do have beneficial effects other than analgesia, such as inducing drowsiness and inducing euphoria in some patients, they act differently on the brain than when they are used inappropriately. The risk of addiction in these circumstances is demonstrably small. It should also be mentioned that, especially in situations of refractory pain that appear to resist treatment, the use of adjuvant analgesics such as anticonvulsant and antidepressant medication can prove effective.

Finally, no consideration of pain would be complete without considering the phenomenon of 'phantom pain'. This occurs in amputees who continue to experience the sensation including extreme pain, from limbs even after they have been removed by amputation. Unfortunately, this pain is very resistant to analgesia and even to the surgical severing of the nerve pathways that transmit pain to the brain at the spinal cord. The theory is that the brain retains an imprint of the limb and the pain which was suffered and, since the pain is no longer treatable at the site, it is hard to treat this pain as it is generated solely in the brain. Knowledge of phantom pain has led to some developments that benefit patients. For example, it is now routine in patients receiving surgery on, for example, the hand or foot to have the nerves higher up the limbs blocked by local anaesthetic in addition to local anaesthetic at the site of the operation or even being rendered unconscious by a general anaesthetic. This has been demonstrated to reduce the sensation of pain from the site of operation after surgery and this may be because the brain has never, in fact, sensed any pain from the affected site due to the nerve block.

Conclusion

This chapter has considered three adverse physiological phenomena: stress, shock and pain that, to a greater or lesser, degree disturb homeostasis. Stress is a physiological response, with psychological consequences, which arises from sustained real or perceived threats to the body. To a certain extent, stress is an adaptive response to environmental challenges but the prolongation of this response has many adverse consequences and has been associated with several disorders such as cardiovascular disease, depression and anxiety. There are several theories of how stress arises in the body and these guide the therapeutic approaches to stress, which range from 'talk therapies' such as counselling to the use of drugs to alleviate anxiety, relax the body and promote sleep in affected individuals. Nurses should be aware of stress in their patients and in their colleagues and can help to alleviate stress through the provision of information, providing time to talk over problems and develop appropriate coping strategies, and where necessary, administering appropriate prescribed medication.

Shock is a life-threatening condition that has several causes but always has a profound effect on the cardiovascular system leading to poor perfusion of tissues and death in extreme circumstances. Nurses should know how to recognise the signs of shock in their patients and how to take appropriate action in order to maintain the vital functions of the body and preserve life.

Pain, in some circumstances, is a physiological response to injury that may prevent further injury. However, pain may also be chronic, without discernable origin, and appear to serve no useful function. Under these circumstances pain significantly reduces the quality of life of the sufferer. Pain is also induced in patients following surgical procedures and, while this is a normal response, its optimal relief is paramount, as pain can slow recovery and lead to respiratory and circulatory problems. The gate control theory of pain is useful in explaining how pain is transmitted to the brain from the peripheries of the body and also how some analgesics and alternative therapies for pain may work. Nurses need to appreciate and understand not only the complexity of pain as an experience and the need for effective assessment, but also the increasingly multimodal means of relieving pain.

Questions

1   Outline the main theories of stress and how these are related to therapeutic approaches to stress.
2   What are the possible adverse consequences of stress on the body?
3   How might shock arise in the body?
4   Describe the stages of shock.
5   How would you recognise shock in someone and what are the first aid actions to be taken if you discover that somebody is in shock?
6   How could you assess pain in a patient?
7   How does the gate control theory of pain contribute to our understanding of pain-relieving measures?
8   Why is it important to alleviate pain in patients post-operatively?

Index